CH

The Montessori Method
for Connecting to
People with Dementia

of related interest

Communication Skills for Effective Dementia Care
A Practical Guide to Communication and Interaction Training (CAIT)
Edited by Ian Andrew James and Laura Gibbons
ISBN 978 1 78592 623 5
eISBN 978 1 78592 624 2

CLEAR Dementia Care©
A Model to Assess and Address Unmet Needs
Dr Frances Duffy
ISBN 978 1 78592 276 3
eISBN 978 1 78450 576 9

**Sharing Sensory Stories and Conversations
with People with Dementia**
A Practical Guide
Joanna Grace
ISBN 978 1 78592 409 5
eISBN 978 1 78450 769 5

Adaptive Interaction and Dementia:
How to Communicate without Speech
Dr Maggie Ellis and Professor Arlene Astell
Illustrated by Suzanne Scott
ISBN 978 1 78592 197 1
eISBN 978 1 78450 471 7

Sensory Modulation in Dementia Care
Assessment and Activities for Sensory-Enriched Care
Tina Champagne
ISBN 978 1 78592 733 1
eISBN 978 1 78450 427 4

The **Montessori Method** for **Connecting** to **People with Dementia**

A Creative Guide to Communication and Engagement in Dementia Care

Tom Brenner
and **Karen Brenner**

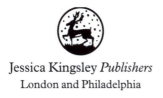

Jessica Kingsley *Publishers*
London and Philadelphia

First published in 2020
by Jessica Kingsley Publishers
73 Collier Street
London N1 9BE, UK
and
400 Market Street, Suite 400
Philadelphia, PA 19106, USA

www.jkp.com

Library of Congress Cataloging in Publication Data
A CIP catalog record for this book is available from the Library of Congress

British Library Cataloguing in Publication Data
A CIP catalogue record for this book is available from the British Library

ISBN 978 1 78592 813 0
eISBN 978 1 78450 873 9

Printed and bound in Great Britain

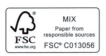

Contents

Acknowledgments 9

1. Introduction: Karen Brenner and Tom Brenner . . . 11

2. Thomas Kitwood and Maria Montessori 25

3. The Past is Another Country 41

4. The Storied Memory 55

5. Dementia and Creativity 75

6. Drum Circles 85

7. Just Sing Your Song 97

8. Poetry Circles 109

9. Video Diaries 127

10. The Lamplighters 139

Endnotes 151

Index 153

This book is dedicated to our family, our children,
and our grandchildren who have all given us
unfailing support and encouragement.

What can you do to promote world peace?
Go home and love your family. (Mother Teresa)

Acknowledgments

We would like to thank all of the wonderful people who were the inspiration for this book, the people living with dementia, and their carers. You have all taught us so much about patience, resilience, joy in the moment, and true grit. Your generosity and brave hearts will forever be an inspiration to us.

We have been further enriched by the professionals we've met along the way. We are very grateful to you for sharing your expertise with us and for contributing so generously to this book. We would like to thank in particular:

Dr. Cameron Camp, who put our feet upon this path and who bravely sang karaoke with us one night in an Ecuadorian bar.

Sitar Rose, who so generously shared her video portraits and taught us the great lesson of being still and deeply listening.

Marilyn Raichle, who very kindly shared her mother's experience of creating art throughout her Alzheimer's journey.

John Killick, whose pioneering work in the field of creativity and dementia, and his wonderful book,

Poetry and Dementia: A Practical Guide, inspired our own elder poetry circles.

Tom Gill and his exuberant drum circles; he teaches all of us how to find joy in the rhythms of life.

The Intergenerational Choir and the Alzheimer Society London and Middlesex, Ontario, Canada, who taught us that we all should find our own songs and sing them!

Chapter One

Introduction: Karen Brenner and Tom Brenner

Karen's story

When I first met him, he was a young man with only two speeds, working flat out or sound asleep. He has been a drummer, a machinist, a medic, and is now a gerontologist. He can repair anything that breaks, from a washing machine to a heart. He is the person who will always, *always,* come to the aid of others. (The American Red Cross honored him in 2010 as Hero of the Year.) He is a wonderful storyteller with a wild streak, a lover of jazz and art. He is also hot-tempered, impatient, opinionated, and demanding, with very high expectations for himself and for others.

That is why I was so shocked the first time I saw him interacting with a person who has dementia. I was so used to the impatient, quick, restless man. Who was this person of patience, quiet, and calm? When he works with people who are living with dementia, he slows everything down, his speech, his movements, and his expectations. He sits quietly with people, waiting patiently for them to form their thoughts, never interrupting, never showing the slightest sign of being bored or restless. His name is Tom, and he is my husband.

Reaching the unreachable

Tom and I began working with people who have dementia 20 years ago. At that time, we had been married for many years, had raised our children, mourned the loss of our parents, and supported each other in our mutual return to graduate school. We had been through a lot. I thought I knew him pretty well after all of these years together and all of the experiences we had shared. I was wrong. I was in for a complete shock when we began working together, building our memory support program.

With his history and his personality, I was expecting Tom to experience a long and difficult learning curve working with people who have dementia. Again, I was wrong. The term "like a duck to water" might have been coined to describe Tom's introduction to the world of dementia. From the first moment, he was perfectly at home, perfectly at ease, perfectly happy working with, talking to, and just being with people who are living with dementia.

There is a kind of magic that happens when Tom begins his work. I have watched him now for years and am still amazed by his ability to reach people. Our memory support program gives Tom (and everyone using it) many tools to interact successfully with people who have dementia. In Tom's hands, these tools become a powerful device to reach people who may seem unreachable.

When we walk into a long-term care home, a memory enhancement center, an adult day care facility, we often meet groups of people who are just sitting, staring into space, seemingly not aware of their surroundings or each other. Tom will sit down with this group and in ten minutes they are talking and laughing, or singing, or playing drums together. I have seen this happen over and over and over for years, and every single time I am moved to tears.

Applying Montessori methods to dementia care

For me, the transition from being a Montessori teacher working with children to interacting with elders was not so easy. I was, quite frankly, frightened of people who had dementia. I grew up in a family for whom scenes of any type were an anathema. The idea of interacting with people who might shout at me or cry or grab me was abhorrent. But Tom had done extensive research on person-centered dementia care and was convinced that the work I was doing with children in a Montessori classroom could be translated into a program for people living with dementia.

I had been working for many years in an inclusion program with children who are deaf. The highly organized, visual, stimulating Montessori environment proved to be perfect for children who couldn't hear and had difficulties in communication. I could intellectually understand the parallels that Tom drew from the prepared environment of the Montessori classroom and a good, person-centered care home. But I was scared.

I well remember the day that I decided I just couldn't do this work with Tom. We had been volunteering at a long-term care home on Saturday afternoons. We would bring in different Montessori materials and exercises to share with the people living in the home. The older people seemed to be drawn to the beautiful materials just as the children were. I could see that Tom was on to something, that there was an obvious interest in the Montessori work. The older people would watch us patiently and then try the work themselves. We introduced flower arranging, flags of the world, fabric matching, any Montessori material that we thought might be helpful and interesting to the people in the care home. But there was one resident who did not like our being there. She would shout at us, tell us to go away, that no one wanted us there, and that we were interfering with people and bothering them. She would raise her arm as if she was going to strike us, but she never did. That didn't matter to me; Bridget really frightened me.

So that Saturday afternoon, as we stood just outside the door of the care home and the autumn leaves swirled around our feet, the cold wind snatching our voices away, I told Tom,

"I don't want to go back today. I'm afraid of some of those people. You know how much I hate scenes and last Saturday Bridget yelled at us again. I just froze when she took off her slipper and started hitting that other woman on the head with it. You knew what to do, how to calm her down. I don't know what I'm doing here. I'm just a Montessori teacher. You're the gerontologist, you're the one who spent the last six years researching this. I'm not going in there, Tom!"

He took my hand.

"Come on, Karen, we're in this thing together. We'll learn how to do this as we go. We're a great team, aren't we? We've been married forever, we've raised great kids, we beat cancer together!"

I shook my head.

"I wasn't as afraid of cancer as I am of Bridget. She hates us."

Tom wouldn't give up.

"We're meant to do this and I can't do it without you."

With that, he pushed open the door to the care home and with his lopsided smile, whispered to me,

"Anyway, Bridget doesn't hate *us*, Bridget hates *you*!"

So you see, I do understand when family members say to us that they don't want to visit their loved ones anymore. We have often heard this lament, "Why should we go visit Mom now? She doesn't even know who we are anymore.

She just sits and stares out the window and we just sit and stare at her."

"We can't be brave by ourselves"

It is heartbreaking and sometimes frightening to be in the presence of a person who knew you intimately and now, seemingly, doesn't have a clue who you are and doesn't seem to care about you. It is only natural to have these feelings, just as it was natural for me to feel embarrassed and disturbed when some of the people we were working with started screaming uncontrollably or throwing things or didn't remember who I was when I had just spent an hour working with them a few minutes ago. We tend to judge this type of behavior as though the person screaming or not remembering has some control over their behavior. Of course they don't. But it's so hard to see a parent or a spouse behave without any control or have them look at you, the person they've known and loved for years, and recoil from you. It took me many months to get up the courage to face this part of dementia, to get past the idea that these were adults who should be able to control themselves.

When we try to communicate with people living with dementia, we often face hostile, angry, frightened or non-communicative people. After a lot of trial and error Tom and I learned that rather than judging the various behaviors we encounter in this work, it is our responsibility to understand what is going on with the person. We must approach each person as an individual, respecting the emotions they display, being mindful of their personal space, making sure we re-introduce ourselves to the person each time we meet with them. When we show this sort of respect to the people we work with and care for, we begin to open up the path to engagement and relationship.

I had learned to deal with children who threw tantrums, who screamed and cried for no apparent reason. Many of these children had no way to tell me what was going on with them. But I had an understanding and an innate sympathy for the children. The adults who threw tantrums or stared right through me, these people frightened and upset me. In the care home where Tom and I first started our work, I met an older woman who helped me understand my role in the world of dementia. When one of the people who lived in the home started yelling and cursing, this older woman saw me begin to back away and knew that I was frightened. She took my hand and told me,

"You don't need to be afraid. We're just people. We know something's wrong, but we don't know what. We're afraid, too, but someone has to be brave."

She patted my hand.

"And it looks like it has to be you because we can't be brave by ourselves."

Her words have never left me. *We can't be brave by ourselves.* It doesn't come easy for me to interact with someone who's angry or hostile but, like so many of you, I've learned to be brave because someone has to be brave, and it looks like it has to be us.

That was the way we began our work in dementia care, digging deep for our courage, learning from our mistakes, finding out what worked, and trying to understand why it worked. We have had the enormous good fortune to meet people with dementia who were kind and patient and generous with us. We've also met lots of "Bridgets," people who were difficult, sometimes violent. We learned from these hard cases that if we didn't give up on them, we could find a way to reach even them.

I first learned about reaching people who may seem unreachable when I spent 20 years working with children who are deaf or communication-disordered. I had no idea that my experiences teaching special needs children in an inclusion program in a Montessori school would lead to working with older people who were struggling with communication and connection. It's strange, isn't it, the circuitous routes we take in life? I believe that if we are living the life we're meant to live, that everything we experience will prove to be very helpful to us as we face new challenges. In this caregiving work there are so many times that we need to call on our own experiences; times past when we had to show great patience or understanding or fortitude. It is as if we were always preparing for this moment, this time in our lives when we would be called upon to gather up every ounce of courage and kindness and sheer grit that we possess.

A personal challenge

Before we began working in the dementia field, I had one of those experiences that called on every ounce of courage and grit that I could muster. Out of the blue, I was diagnosed with uterine cancer. Once the news was delivered, it seemed as though life moved at warp speed. In only a few days, I was in hospital for major surgery and facing a long, difficult recovery. One week I was living my life and the next week, I was in a hospital bed hooked up to machines and feeling like I was starring in someone else's movie. How did this happen to me? How did I end up here?

Without realizing it, I began to face cancer by using my Montessori training. I isolated the difficulty of each day; sometimes, it was each hour. I coped with the daunting task of fighting cancer and regaining my health by breaking each difficulty down into very small steps. I would think only of the step in front of me. I even used the image of a car's headlights, lighting up only that little bit of road in front of me. Of course, my family, friends, and doctors were most instrumental in pulling me through and putting my feet on the path to recovery. It wasn't until sometime later that I realized how I had used my Montessori training to face the challenges of a health crisis. This story is to illustrate that the Montessori Method is a philosophy that can guide us through the entirety of our lives. It is based on common-sense guidelines and the core belief that we must believe and trust in ourselves and in others. The Montessori philosophy is rooted in finding the strength and abilities of each person. Surviving cancer, I found strength that I didn't know I possessed. I am very grateful for all the gifts that Dr. Montessori has given me. Supplying a road map for surviving cancer is one of the very best gifts of all!

I am also very grateful to the medical professionals and my family and friends who cared for me while I was recovering from cancer. Being a carer is a noble calling but it is also often a lonely one. We humans have a deep-seated need to communicate with each other. If we cannot share our feelings, ideas, ourselves with others, we can become very frustrated and isolated. We've seen this happen to older people who are living with dementia. They lose their ability to use language and so they lash out or withdraw. Children who have communication problems behave much the same way. With both populations, it is vital to believe that we can find some way to reach them and to help them find some way to reach us.

Building on strengths

I was fortunate to meet a little boy who taught me the lesson of never giving up on people who may seem unreachable. A young couple who had just recently immigrated to America from Eastern Europe came to the Montessori school where I was teaching. The mother had in her arms her three-year-old boy. He was limp, disengaged, withdrawn. His mother began to cry when she told me that the doctors said her boy would never be anything more than a vegetable. Her son had contracted meningitis and the high fever and illness had damaged his brain. I reached out and touched her son's hand. He looked up at me and I saw something in his eyes, a spark of interest, a liveliness. I told his parents that we would work with their son, but I made no promises.

I worked with their little boy for three years. It was often one step forward, two steps back. Sometimes I despaired, sometimes he despaired, but we soldiered on. There was something there, something in his eyes that made me want to try harder, to find a way to reach him. Three years later, when he was six years old, I sat with him as he read a book aloud to me, those bright eyes of his following the text, stopping occasionally to look up at me and smile.

My years working with special needs children taught me that we should never give up on people who are struggling to communicate. We know that life can be difficult and frustrating for people living with dementia and the people who love them; it is our mission to discover and build on the remaining strengths and spared abilities of elders. We recognize and work with the limitations that dementia imposes on them, but we look for that spark, that moment when they are with us again; even if just for a fleeting minute, we are once again connected.

Connection

Martin Buber, the well-known philosopher, wrote that once we interact with a place, or a thing, or a person, those things and that person and we ourselves are forever changed.[1] The most simple of meetings, just a discussion of the weather or a stranger smiling at us on the street can change our outlook on the day or the place. Buber wrote that there are two types of exchanges we engage in every day. One is the "I–It" meeting. It is how a person views the world. The other common exchange Buber called the "I–Thou" meeting. Just by having a simple conversation, by simply talking to one another, we can be forever changed, or perhaps, forever change another person. We've all had the experience of feeling down in the dumps and then someone, perhaps a complete stranger, someone we pass on the street, or a clerk at a shop, will smile at us or say something kind to us and suddenly the sun is shining and our whole day looks different. Understanding what Buber is saying is vital to our caregiving work. We need to be deeply aware that our attitude, the way we greet the people we care for, can make a huge difference to the way the day goes. But this isn't a one-way street. If our smile and our positive attitude can uplift the elders we care for, they can also create a better day for us by being kind and patient with us. The simplest exchange can lead to the most profound moment of connection and joy.

This is what our book is all about, learning how to reach and stay connected to people who are living with dementia. All of the techniques and strategies in this book have been field tested by us. We know they work because we've seen it happen with our own eyes! We will share many of the stories and experiences of our work in the field to illustrate the various techniques we use to communicate and connect with elders. These strategies are all accessible and designed to be used by carers who always have limited time and often low reserves of energy. We are writing this book so that you can open it at any page and find something that will be of help to you in a very down-to-earth practical way, or will give you that bit of hope and inspiration needed to get you through the difficult days and the anxious nights. It is our most heartfelt wish that you will find our program to be of real value to you as accessible, vibrant, and practical, which will lead to moments of connectedness, and of joy and of love.

Tom's story

As a young man, it never occurred to me that I would devote much of my life to working with people who have dementia. My youth was largely devoted to playing jazz, blues, and rock and roll. My dream was to become a writer for *Downbeat*, the definitive magazine for jazz aficionados and musicians. I also experienced hard physical labor, working in factories in Chicago to pay for my tuition at university. But then I opened a letter from the US government, greetings from Uncle Sam, telling me that the US Army required my service. I received excellent training as a combat medic, and suddenly my goals were narrowed down to one very simple one, staying alive.

I came very close to not fulfilling this goal on a warm night in November while on guard duty. I was shot three times, the bullets missing my aorta and spine by centimeters and one bullet lodging in my gut. The surgical team that saved my life was headed up by a tough colonel with the stump of a cigar in his teeth, shouting orders to his crew. I remained conscious for the X-rays, the visit from a priest, all the preliminaries before I went under the knife. I remember feeling absolute fury that some faceless attacker thought he had the right to take my life. And there was this red-headed girl who was waiting for me to come home.

I am telling you about my experience of being the victim of violence for only one reason: I have battled post-traumatic stress disorder (PTSD) from the time I was injured in the military until this very day. My psychological problems wax and wane but never truly leave me. I know what it means to wake up in the middle of the night, mind racing, feeling anxious, vulnerable, unsure of where I am. I know what it feels like to be uncomfortable in social situations, to feel trapped, to feel frightened, to lose confidence in my judgment, to wonder if what I am feeling is real or imagined. I don't have dementia, but I have a very good understanding of what the dementia experience is like for those living through it and for those who love them.

I also understand that I am a very lucky man. I survived terrible injuries and went on to marry that red-headed girl and have children and now grandchildren. But I still have to find a way to cope with PTSD every day and every night. There is no simple answer for this condition, no magic pill, just as there is no simple solution for dementia. There is, however, help for me and my fellow veterans who have been diagnosed with PTSD and there is help for those who have been diagnosed with dementia. Studying the Montessori Method, both its application and philosophy, has helped me learn to cope in more productive ways with my PTSD. The Montessori Method has also helped me in some ways that I could never have anticipated.

Applying the Montessori philosophy

The Montessori philosophy can be applied in all aspects of our lives. Here is an example: One of the members of my family became a hoarder. She inherited the family home and spent years trashing it. It became my mission to clean and pack up the house for sale when she moved out. The first time I entered the house I had to don a hazmat (decontamination) suit. It was a heartbreaking chore, emotionally and physically draining. From my understanding of the Montessori Method I knew that any task, whether simple or daunting, is approached by isolating the difficulty and breaking the job down into simple steps. So, instead of facing the seemingly impossible chore of sorting out a large, destroyed home, I began by facing one corner of one room. I cleaned that corner, threw away some things, cleaned and packed others. That is how this wrecked house was eventually cleaned and sorted, one small area at a time.

When you are looking at your life as a carer, we ask you to face this enormous task by breaking it down into small steps, isolating each difficulty. We are here to help you find solutions to the difficulty of reaching and staying connected to the person or people you are caring for. This is my life goal now: finding accessible tools that will assist carers in staying connected to people living with dementia. This is why Karen and I are writing this book, and why we've spent the last 20 years working directly with people diagnosed with dementia. People who have dementia are the same people they always have been, only now they have to cope with certain difficulties, challenges, and limitations.

As noted earlier, many of us have some form of psychological, physical, or emotional challenges in our lives. We usually find strategies, some form of coping mechanisms to make it through our days, even with our personal difficulties. Now, we must find strategies to face the exhaustive times we face as carers. We believe that it is incumbent on those of us who are carers to find those accommodations, those aids necessary to make life with dementia less lonely, less frightening, less confusing, for both the carer and for those they love and care for.

One of the strategies we have found to be very helpful in this caregiving journey is to try and change the way we think about dementia and to consider our role of caregiver in a different light. What if we begin to think of dementia as a disability and not a disease? What if we begin to create proactive accommodations for people living with dementia? Can we make their lives more successful, more integrated into society, more joyful? We will demonstrate many strategies and techniques in this book that can do just that!

We also want to help you find those small moments of victory that do exist in caregiving, even if it is just a fleeting smile or a squeeze of the hand. These are moments to be celebrated and treasured, these are the small moments that can help carry us through the rough times. We want to give you the tools so that you can recreate your connection to the person who has dementia, to help you establish new inroads to reach them. Communication, compassion, connection—this is our life's passion. This is our beginning point. This is our goal now.

Chapter Two

Thomas Kitwood and Maria Montessori

Dr. Thomas Kitwood's story

Today, it is very common to hear the term "person-centered care." It is used by professionals in the field of caregiving as well as those who design intentional homes and adult day centers. But what, exactly, does person-centered care mean? Thomas Kitwood is considered by many to be the father of person-centered dementia care.

Dr. Kitwood was ordained as a priest at Wycliffe Hall in 1962. After completing his National Service, he moved to Uganda to teach chemistry at Busoga Boys School, where he also became school chaplain. From this experience, Dr. Kitwood wrote his first book in 1970, *What is Human?* He returned to the UK and was awarded a PhD in Social Psychology at the University of Bradford in 1977.

It was at the University of Bradford that Dr. Kitwood founded Bradford Dementia Group, the organization that pioneered and advanced the idea of person-centered dementia care. The method was considered revolutionary because it took the viewpoint of the person with dementia. Simply put, person-centered dementia care means that we try and look at each situation through the eyes of the person we care for. In his groundbreaking 1997 book,

Dementia Reconsidered: The Person Comes First,[2] Dr. Kitwood carefully lays out the explanation of person-centered dementia care, how to use it, and why it is vital for the wellbeing of both the cared for and the caregiver.

In the three-day training course that Dr. Kitwood created, he taught the concept of dementia care mapping. This is a tool to help caregivers understand the flow of activity and behavioral patterns of someone living with dementia. It is essential for caregivers to understand what they are seeing, and to be able to discern what they are observing. This is not easy, of course, but if we can try and implement the objectives defined by Dr. Kitwood, the lives of the people we care for and our own lives will become much less combative, much more peaceful, much more connected.

Dementia Care Mapping was created by Dr. Tom Kitwood to provide an observational tool that is at once objective and yet sensitive to patterns of behavior and the unique needs of the individual being observed. The results of the observations of the qualified Dementia Care Mapper is shared with the staff so that they can implement a care program that meets the needs of the person.

Dr. Maria Montessori's story

Dr. Maria Montessori also believed in putting the person first. She based an entire educational system, method, and philosophy on the belief that a school should serve the needs of the child.[3]

Rome, 1896: a beautiful and valiant young woman became the first female to earn a medical degree in Italy. She studied not only medicine, but had also been to engineering school, and exhaustively researched the education systems of the day. Later, she would embark on the pursuit of a PhD in Anthropology. Maria Montessori was not welcome at the medical school in Rome. She was considered to be uncouth and ill mannered for pursuing a medical degree, as women were not supposed to be exposed to diseases, injuries, and naked bodies. Maria was ignored by her professors and spat upon by her fellow medical students. She was forced to dissect cadavers alone at night in the basement of the medical school because it was not considered proper for a woman to be in the presence of men when dissecting a naked body. All alone with the cadavers, she sang opera very loudly, and very badly, to allay her fears, and smoked cigarettes to cover the smell of formaldehyde. She persisted in her medical studies and won awards for her work.

Dr. Montessori's first professional assignment was to care for the children who were housed in an insane asylum in Rome. Some of these children's parents were patients in the asylum and some of the children had been diagnosed with learning disabilities. There was no educational program for these children; they were not even allowed to go outside to play. The very first thing that Dr. Montessori did with the children was to take them outside to dance in the rain.

Using materials

Dr. Montessori used the observational skills she had acquired in medical school to carefully observe the children in her care. She saw the children scrabbling on the floor after meals, picking up scraps of the food that fell from the table, and rolling it around and around in their hands. The staff were disgusted by this behavior, but Dr. Montessori understood that the children needed something useful, something meaningful to do with their hands. She used her engineering skills to build beautiful, well-crafted materials that the children could manipulate with their hands. Each material taught a different skill, isolating one difficulty at a time. The materials were created with a built-in control of error so that there was only one way to successfully use them. This allowed the people using Montessori materials to explore and discover on their own. Dr. Montessori was one of the first educators to understand that people of all ages learn best by doing, by interacting with tools that teach one concept at a time. In the Montessori Method, people are allowed to work with the materials for as long as they wish.

Memory systems: procedural and declarative

The children were captivated by the materials that Montessori created for them. She found that after she demonstrated how to use an exercise, the children would often work with the same material over and over again. Allowing the children to work with each material repetitively called into use the procedural memory system, sometimes referred to as implicit or muscle memory. This memory system gives people the ability to instantly retrieve procedural memories to complete processes like reading a book or tying shoes. It is a form of long-term memory and can be included in the sub-category of implicit memory. The memory is created by constant practice of a skill until the neural systems are able to perform the task on autopilot. The procedural memory system tends to be the memory system that is the least affected by dementia. This is one of the reasons that the Montessori approach to dementia care is so successful and effective. We tap into the procedural memory system, building our program around exercises and activities that use repetitive muscle movement.

There is another type of memory system that tends to be more affected by dementia: the declarative memory.

Declarative memory is fact-based and refers to those memories that can be consciously recalled or declared. This includes facts such as the name of the President of the United States, how many inches in one foot, the day's date or a loved one's name. Declarative memory is a subset of explicit memory, those memories that are explicitly stored and are consciously recalled. It is also the memory system that is responsible for episodic memory (remembering an event or a date) and semantic memory (remembering someone's name or the names of common objects). Executive function is also considered a subset of the declarative or explicit memory system. It is what we use when we're planning a trip, deciding where to have lunch, or trying to choose which career path we should explore. It helps us make small, large, and life-changing decisions. The declarative memory system is the system that tends to be most negatively impacted by dementia. That is why it is common for people living with dementia to forget common facts, to forget that they just ate lunch and sadly, to forget the names of people they love.

We often remind carers (both professional and family carers) that this type of forgetting is part of the condition of dementia. Although it doesn't take away the hurt when someone's mother doesn't remember their name, if we take the time to understand declarative memory and how it is impacted by dementia, we can begin to take this sort of forgetting less personally. We encourage carers to understand that, while the person with dementia may not remember your name, they still love and care for you. In our work, we have found that trying to stay away from the declarative memory system (facts, dates, episodes) and concentrating more on facilitating the use of the procedural or muscle memory provides a much more successful interaction. The Montessori approach to person-centered dementia care is based on the use of this muscle memory.

Dr. Montessori found that children learn best by doing, by working with the materials she created for them. The children were encouraged to work with these materials for as long as they wanted. Dr. Montessori understood that working on a task repetitively created long-lasting muscle memories. Because Dr. Montessori created a learning system built on the procedural memory system, the children in her schools learned math sensorially, through their bodies. They learned to read by tracing sandpaper letters with their fingertips over and over. They learned geography by tracing the continents and then drawing them free hand. It is important to understand the central role that the procedural memory system plays in the Montessori Method so that we can build exercises and activities for elders based on muscle memory.

A prepared environment

Because Dr. Montessori had such great success working with the children in the asylum in Rome, she was asked to start a school for children in the infamous San Lorenzo slums. On January 6, 1907, the Casa dei Bambini (Children's House) was opened and the first Montessori school was born. Dr. Montessori realized that the children living in the San Lorenzo slums desperately needed a place where they could feel safe and secure, a space that met their needs and piqued their interests. With this in mind, she created an environment built strictly on the needs of the children. Dr. Montessori was one of the pioneers in the creation of child-sized furniture. She hung paintings at eye level for the children (not the teachers). The Casa dei Bambini was prepared to fit the needs of the children: their need to move, their need for order, their need for beauty, their need for living things in the environment (plants and animals). Dr. Montessori wanted to bring the world to the children of the San Lorenzo slums.

Dr. Montessori's idea of creating a prepared environment to meet the needs of the people using it has been adopted by the person-centered care movement. Today, progressive long-term care homes, adult day centers, and memory cafes all support the belief that these intentional communities must be designed and created to fulfill the needs of the elders using them. Enlightened person-centered care communities put the person with dementia in the center of the care program. The physical design of the space must provide for elders who may need extra space for walkers and wheelchairs. Furniture is chosen that is comfortable, sturdy, and easy to get into and out of. Carpets and wall coverings should have no design, or a very simple design. Communities for elders can be made more home-like by bringing in animals and plants that the community members can care for and enjoy. All of these ideas about person-centered care communities seem quite familiar to us now. This prepared environment movement that began in a little school in the San Lorenzo slums of Rome in 1907 was eventually adapted for elders by Dr. Thomas Kitwood in the late 1970s.

Independent learners

Along with creating an environment prepared for the children, Dr. Montessori began to develop a curriculum designed to give her students opportunities to become independent learners. She observed that when children were allowed to care for their environment, to make choices, to solve their own disputes peacefully, to have the opportunity to practice compassion, they began to learn and grow without struggle and without strife. Throughout her long career, Dr. Montessori always insisted that she did not create the Montessori Method; the children did. She observed them and they taught her what they needed to fulfill their work of becoming independent, productive, and caring people. Today, there are thousands of Montessori schools in 122 countries. Dr. Montessori traveled throughout the world, creating training centers for Montessori teachers and establishing schools for children from birth to 18 years of age.

Common ground

We have introduced you to Thomas Kitwood and Maria Montessori because they are the founders of the methodologies that we use in our work in dementia care. Here is a summation of the common ground that Thomas Kitwood and Maria Montessori share:

- The Montessori approach to dementia care and Kitwood's person-centered care for dementia both teach that the *environment should serve the needs of the people using it*. For elders living in either an intentional community or a family home, safety is, of course, the number one concern. The environment should be free of clutter and, if possible, carpets and wallpaper should be simple, with little or no design on them— carpets with swirls or lines can be confusing and can lead to falls. Plants and animals, when practical, bring points of interest and comfort, especially in more institutional settings. Everything—carpeting, furniture, paintings, temperature, lighting—needs to be carefully considered with the specialized needs of the people using the environment. For example, if the tablecloths, napkins, and plates are all the same color, it might be difficult for people to differentiate these objects. Some homes and adult day centers use contrasting colored toilet seats to distinguish the seat from the rest of the white toilet. As with all aspects of person-centered dementia care, we need to take time to consider all aspects of the environment, making sure that the setting meets the needs of the people using it.

- Kitwood and Montessori both created *strength-based philosophies*. In dementia care, this means looking for and maintaining the spared abilities and remaining strengths of the individual. These strengths may be that a person has a wonderful smile, or they are able to read aloud to others, or they have a beautiful singing voice, or they know a lot of jokes. When we take the time to really look, we can find the strengths and spared abilities of people living with dementia. We can build on this knowledge and create exercises and activities that support these remaining strengths.

- Both Kitwood and Montessori *recognize and honor the child that lives within all of us*, no matter our age. It is often said that people with dementia are childish or that they return to their childhood. While it is true that their memories of childhood may be more intact than their memories of the present day, this doesn't mean that people who have dementia are like children. The Montessori Method encourages carers to treat people who have dementia with the respect and dignity they deserve as our elders. Calling people with dementia pet names or being affectionate with them without their permission can make them very uncomfortable. It is important to be genuine and to care deeply about the people we care for, but it is equally important to be respectful of both their space and their sense of self.

- Kitwood and Montessori stress *care for the whole person*: the physical, emotional, and spiritual needs of the individual. This concept seems so basic on the face of it. Of course we're going to care for the whole person, but in reality, consistently making this happen is very challenging. Carers are often exhausted taking care of the first part of this equation, the physical wellbeing of someone living with dementia. This is a huge responsibility and often takes up the lion's share of the caregiving day. How can there be time and energy to also care for a person's emotional and spiritual needs? If we are mindful, we can find moments where we can support the emotional and spiritual needs of people too. Sometimes, it can be as simple as listening intently for a minute or two, or we can watch a beautiful sunset together, or listen to a much loved piece of music. If we look for them, there are opportunities for us to tend to emotional and spiritual needs as we also care for physical needs.

- Both Montessori and Kitwood emphasize *identifying and meeting individual needs in care plans and/or educational plans*. The medical field recognizes that everyone's journey through dementia is unique. As far as we are able, we should try to tailor the Montessori program to fit the needs of each person. We can gather information from care staff and family members.

What was the person really passionate about? What did they love to do for hobbies or for fun? Then we can bring in objects from these areas of interest. Families and friends can be enormously helpful in this area.

- Both methods can *bring order out of chaos* (whether the chaos is in the environment or within the person). In implementing the Montessori Method for positive dementia care, we have observed that when people are engaged in meaningful exercises and activities, the frequency of bouts of agitation and acting out go down precipitously. We all need a reason to get up in the morning; we all need to feel productive and needed. That is the motivation for creating this program: we give elders opportunities to be productive again and engaged in meaningful work. In these ways, they are again connected to their world. This connection may last for a day, an hour, or five minutes, but when it happens, it's magic.

- People applying these methods benefit from the acknowledgment that the *individualized needs of the carer are recognized and respected*: "Create a care setting in which feelings are experienced and expressed and where people have permission to ask for support when they feel they need it."[4] If we don't take care of ourselves (both professional and family carers), then we cannot help anyone else. Just as the person with dementia is on their own unique journey, so are the people who care for them. As you look for ways to comfort and strengthen the person you care for, you need to look just as hard for those things that bring you rest and rejuvenation. Everyone needs support during these caregiving days. Everyone! Remember that when you ask someone else for help, you're giving them the opportunity to be in a state of grace. There is no greater gift than giving help and support to those in need, whether that person is a family caregiver, a friend, or a professional carer.

- The *use of positive language* is essential to the success of both methods:[5] "Everything you say to another person is absorbed, catalogued and remembered." It takes a conscious effort to use positive language with the people we are caring for. Even the most benign negative comment can create anxiety and tension in the person with dementia. For example, instead of saying, "But you must remember Mary. She lived next door to us for 40 years!" you could change this to a much more positive exchange by saying, "Oh, here's Mary. She lived next door to us and always loved your apple pie." Choosing positive language isn't always easy, but this one change can make a huge difference in interactions with the people we care for.

- There is another aspect of language that is important to discuss because it can be challenging to achieve. When talking with people who have dementia, we should *try to drop the word "remember" from our vocabulary*. When we're having a conversation, we often, without thinking, say to the other person, "Don't you remember…?" If we ask the person with dementia to try and remember something, we're giving them an impossible task, and possibly setting up feelings of agitation and anxiety. We recognize that it is very difficult to drop the word "remember," but it is essential that we try. In the same vein, we should also *refrain from asking the person with dementia to answer direct questions about factual information*. When we first began this work, we would be so enthusiastic about our discussions that we would often ask questions like, "How long were you married?" or "Where were you living then?" In response, we would get the thousand-mile stare as an answer to our question. Over time we learned that asking for facts (time, place, event, name, etc.) only served to stop the discussion cold. We know how difficult it is, but we also know how important it is to use positive language, to forget the word "remember," and never ask for facts when having conversations with people living with dementia.

- Kitwood and Montessori ask us to *give the people we work with choices whenever possible*. This concept of the invitation is central to the Montessori Method. We invite; we never insist that people join our work We have observed that sometimes when a person declines to work with us, they will still watch what we are doing. Or there are times when people say they don't want to join us and then they see other people having fun and they decide to join in. When people do join in, we employ the Montessori maxim: follow the person. The exercise we've set up may be a word-finding game. Often, the participants are more interested in having a discussion about one of the words than playing the game. We will follow the person or group and allow them to take the discussion wherever they want it to go.

    There is a phenomenon in dementia known as "failure to initiate." This difficulty in beginning a task or a conversation may stem from the impact dementia has on executive function (the ability to make large and small decisions). While we always respect the person's right to choose or to say no, we need to be mindful of the phenomenon of *failure to initiate*. We can wait patiently and encourage people to participate, trying to help them overcome their doubts and fears but, in the end, we must allow for choice. The people we work with have lived long and, most likely, productive lives, and we should honor this by giving them choices as often as possible. These can be as simple as which toothpaste to use or where they want to sit to have lunch. By giving people choices throughout their day (always taking into account the need for health and safety) we honor their dignity and help them maintain their ability to connect to their environment.

- The concept of *empathetic identification* is essential to both methods: carers are encouraged to strive to see the world as those they serve see the world. Simply put, this concept means that we should slow down our pace to match the pace of the people we are caring for. We should anticipate, as much as possible, the difficulties they may have with a task and try to bypass the difficulty when we can. Looking for signs of pain or discomfort is also part of empathetic identification. We can brighten a person's day by attending to small matters that may loom large in their lives—cleaning their eye glasses to make sure there are no smudges, making sure that hearing aids are turned on and working properly, checking clothing to see if everything fits properly, making sure that the person isn't too hot or too cold. Taking care of the small things can make everyone's day much better.

Dr. Kitwood and Dr. Montessori believed passionately in the probity and beauty of the human spirit. Because our program is rooted in these two philosophies, we strive to create and maintain an honest, compassionate, and effective program for people living with dementia and their carers. Both Thomas Kitwood and Maria Montessori were pioneers in their respective fields, building programs that were revolutionary for their time, and creating positive cultural changes, both in dementia care and education.

We believe that it is important to know the history of the Montessori Method in order to better understand why we use this approach in our work. We find the synchronicity of the Montessori Method and Kitwood's approach to be an essential part of our program.

The person at the center

Keeping the person with dementia at the center of a care program may seem like an easy thing to do, but in reality it takes a conscious, determined effort to see the world through their eyes and to respond accordingly. When you think about it, this is the only approach that makes complete sense. The person with dementia can't make changes to the way they are living, just as children cannot change the circumstances of the life that the adults around them provide. Both of these populations are vulnerable and dependent. Children, it is hoped, will go on to live independent and responsible lives, whereas elders cannot have that expectation. However, we can (and we do) give the people we care for opportunities to be as independent as they can be for as long as they can. One of the unique and powerful aspects of our use of the Montessori Method is that we provide elders with opportunities to contribute to their families and the wider community. In the following chapters, we will demonstrate how we go about this.

There are so many parallels between the Montessori Method and Kitwood's approach: both call on us to use careful observation; both believe in establishing environments that serve the people using them; both honor the spirit of the people we are serving (children and elders); both teach the value of positive language; and both believe in the dignity and beauty of the human being, whether that person is three or eighty-three.

When we strive to do good work (no matter what type of work it is) we know that we all stand on the shoulders of giants. We are humbled and grateful to be carrying forth the work begun by both Dr. Tom Kitwood and Dr. Maria Montessori. Although these two pioneers of care never met, there is a very real kinship between their world views, philosophies, and approach to caring for our elders and for our children.

The child is father of the man. (William Wordsworth)[6]

Chapter Three

The Past is Another Country

One of the most heartbreaking phrases we hear in our caregiving work is: *I want to go home!* We have observed carers trying to find all sorts of solutions to this constant refrain. Sometimes the carer or family member or visiting friend will say something like, "But you sold your house." Or they might say, "You are home. This is your home now." Or well-meaning loved ones and carers might promise to take the person with dementia home later that day, the reasoning being that the person with dementia won't remember the promise to take them home and, for the moment, this promise seems to calm them down.

All of the above responses to the phrase *I want to go home!* are doubtless well intentioned and often spoken with love and concern. But none address the deeper problem: what does a person with dementia really mean when they tell us they want to go home? For some people, this phrase may mean that they want to return to their childhood home. For others, it may mean that they want to return to the home they created for their spouse and children. Within these heartbreaking words there lies a clue to the entire dementia experience. For anyone who has ever experienced a tragedy, a life-changing illness, injury, or unexpected loss, there is a deep-seated longing for life to return to normal. There is a yearning for the life they knew before everything changed forever. We believe that this desire for life to be as it once was is the deeper meaning behind the words *I want to go home!*

But none of us can return to the past. As L.P. Hartley wrote, "The past is a foreign country, they do things differently there."[7] This quotation is important to the discussion at hand because within it are found the clues of how to address this heartbreaking dilemma. The life lived before the onset of dementia is a foreign country and things were done much differently there. Knowing that there is a longing for the past, we can use this knowledge to explore the person's past life. This can be an effective strategy since long-term memory is often more intact than short-term memory for people who live with dementia. For example, we can ask these sorts of open-ended questions:

- What did your childhood bedroom/house/school look like?

- What sort of chores did you have to do at home?

- What did you and your friends do for fun?

- What was your favorite meal?

These kinds of open-ended questions can lead to discussions of life before dementia. Of course, we don't pepper these questions at people; we use open-ended questions carefully to help people remember their earlier lives, and to ease them into warm and comfortable memories.

Putting something meaningful into someone's hands

A powerful tool that we find to be so helpful in helping people connect to both the past and the present is a very simple one: *we put something meaningful in a person's hands* ("meaningful" is the operative word here). We ask the staff and family members to tell us what the person with dementia is interested in, what were their passions, what did they love? With this information we can develop a program that is tailored to that specific person. A man may have been an accountant in his working life but his real love was trains. With this knowledge we can create a simple but powerful program. We could begin with something as basic as handing the person a toy train, or setting up a small train to run on tracks on a table top. These sort of tactile and visual prompts can open the door for many wonderful conversations. It is very important to remember that the Montessori Method encourages us to follow the person and to give the person space and time to talk about their memories. We are guides to help people explore their own lives. We are not the Master of Ceremonies or the arbiters of the truth; we are there to elicit connection and to listen deeply.

Listening deeply

Listening deeply is a skill that should be practiced with a great deal of care and conscious deliberation. It is important to learn how to find the meaning behind the words that are spoken. We should observe body language and voice inflection. We can listen for the nugget of important information that may lie hidden within the language.

The following is an example of how deep listening can play out.

HELEN'S STORY

We were visiting Helen in a long-term care center. While we were there, Helen's son came for a visit. He walked in just as she was in the middle of telling us a story that she had repeated to us several times during this visit. The son sat down and glanced over at us, shaking his head as his mother launched once again into the same story. Her son interrupted her, saying to us,

"See, this is why I hate to come visit her. She says the same things over and over again."

Helen didn't seem too bothered by her son's criticism as she began the same story yet again.

Here is the story that Helen told repeatedly:

"I was a single mother back then and I had to work two jobs. Sometimes my brother would call me up and say, 'Sis, get your butt over here and have some dinner.'" Helen's face would light up with a big smile as she quoted her brother. It seemed such a non-sequitur, this little story, popping up in the middle of a discussion of the weather or meal times. Once Helen started telling this story, she would get into the "dementia loop" and retell it over and over.

When Helen finished telling this story for about the fifth time that day, we asked her this question,

"How did it make you feel, Helen, when your brother invited you over for dinner?"

She looked up at us in surprise, her bright, blue eyes suddenly filling with tears. She answered,

"It made me happy! I was so lonely."

The room went very quiet and then Helen's son walked over to her, hugged her and said,

"I'm sorry, Mom. I didn't know you were lonely."

Helen's son realized that there was a reason his mom was telling this story over and over. He finally heard the important message his mother was trying to convey to him, that she was lonely. Sometimes, it just takes the right question to unlock the meaning behind the words. As Paul Tillich, the German-American philosopher and theologian wrote, "The first duty of love is to listen."

We have experienced many of these breakthrough moments when the meaning behind the words becomes clear. Sometimes, though, it is very difficult to understand what a person with dementia is trying to tell us. The following is an example of how hard this can be in practice.

We were having tea in a local tea shop when the owner of the shop walked over to us, and said, "You saved my life!"

She had overheard a conversation we were having in her tea shop a few weeks earlier with a friend who was asking for our help with her parent who had dementia. We told our friend that even the most nonsensical of statements can have a meaning and purpose if we just take the time to try and figure it out. The owner of the tea shop told us that she was one of the carers for her mother who was living with dementia. She told us this story:

"I told my mother that I would pick her up early for Easter Mass. I suggested that we attend the eight a.m. service instead of our usual nine-thirty mass. I thought that if we went early we could avoid the big crowds and it would be easier for my mom. But Mom looked alarmed and told me that she didn't want to go to that Mass because we might run into bad policemen. I was dumbfounded! I tried to question my mother, asking her about the bad policemen and why she thought they'd be at the earlier Mass. She couldn't answer me and I saw that she was getting very upset and seemed afraid. Then I remembered what I heard you two telling your friend, that it was important to look for the meaning behind the words. Suddenly, I realized that Mom was frightened because I was changing her Sunday morning routine and that upset her. So I told her that we would attend our regular Mass at nine-thirty and she immediately calmed down. She just couldn't handle the change in her routine."

The tea shop owner could have become embroiled in an argument with her mother, trying to dissuade her that there would be no bad policemen at the later Mass, but she realized that it was the emotion her mother was trying to convey to her, not the actual story. So why couldn't her mom just say, "I'm anxious about changing my routine"? This would make the caregiving life so much easier, but most of the time, we're left having to guess, decipher, or intuit what the people we care for are trying to tell us. Sometimes, we get it right. Other times, we're completely lost, but the important thing is to *try and find the meaning behind the words*, even if sometimes we get it wrong.

We happened to get it right one time when we were working with a group of veterans in a long-term care home. We brought with us small squares of matching pairs of different kinds of wood: oak, maple, walnut, cherry, etc. There were about 20 different pairs of small wooden squares. Our idea was that this group of men could match the different squares of wood and it might lead to a conversation about building, woodworking, or perhaps different types of trees. To our surprise, one of the men told the group that this pair of walnut squares looked like the type of wood used for the gun stocks in the Second World War. He proceeded to talk to the group about his time in the army during the war. Other men in the group then joined in the conversation, sharing memories of the

Korean War and the war in Vietnam. Some of the men in the group shed tears. There was laughter and groans and, for a few precious minutes, a real sense of comradery. These men were of different ages, different backgrounds, and in different stages of dementia, but those little wooden squares brought them together and opened their hearts to each other.

The natural world

Another important aspect of the Montessori approach to dementia care is *the role that the natural world plays in helping us connect to people living with dementia and helping them connect to their world*. Dr. Bill Thomas, in his programs for long-term care, The Eden Alternative® and the Green House Project,[1] uses plants and animals to reach people with dementia. He encourages carers to engage elders in the care of these living things by have them water the plants, and feed and groom the animals.

We can bring the outside world to people living in an intentional community by bringing plants and animals into their environment. We can encourage them to garden and to arrange flowers for their common environments, such as dining rooms or living rooms. We can also do very simple things to share the natural world with the people for whom we care. We can bring in a cup of snow for them to feel or a basket of autumn leaves to examine or large smooth stones to hold (making sure the stones are too large to fit into their mouth). We've created a table top Japanese garden with miniature rakes for people to make patterns in the sand.

---

1   www.edenalt.org and https://changingaging.org/the-green-house-project

This simple exercise of quietly raking sand can be very calming and meditative for someone who is feeling agitated.

We were working in a long-term care home, training the staff, and interacting directly with the residents who had dementia. Two of the staff members came up with a wonderful exercise. They put sand in a large baking sheet with high sides and then heated the sand in the oven. When the sand became warm (not hot) they hid small shells in the sand and then asked the residents if they would like to look for the shells. The warm sand felt wonderful to the older people, and finding the beautiful shells brought back memories of holidays by the sea. This simple and beautiful exercise brought so much pleasure and unlocked so many great conversations.

At an adult day center we were being assisted by a young man who was a PhD candidate in Psychology. It was Veterans Day and we brought with us several small US flags to use as prompts for the veterans we were meeting with that day. The young man became very alarmed and asked what we would do if these flags prompted flashbacks of terrible memories or created a lot of agitation for the veterans. We reassured him that if someone became upset we would immediately stop the program and redirect to some other activity.

We handed out the small flags and the veterans began waving them and smiling. One of the older men said that the flags were wrong. He said that there were the wrong number of stars on them. The group then decided to count the number of stars. After finding that there were the correct number of stars on the flag, the group then decided to try and remember all of the names of the states. We began to write the names of the states down on a blackboard in the room as the men called out the different states. As this was going on, different individuals would tell the group about a vacation in this state or having a brother who lived in that state. The conversation was lively and animated, with everyone participating.

We originally thought that when we gave the veterans the flags they might want to sing patriotic songs or talk about their experiences while in the service. Who could have possibly guessed that the flags would turn into a geography lesson with memories of different states shared in the conversation? So, while we hand people with dementia objects that are meaningful or objects from nature, it is important to let them take the conversation and the memories wherever they want to go.

Putting something meaningful in a person's hands is a simple, powerful and accessible technique for helping people with dementia connect to both their past and their present. It is a highly effective way to elicit conversation and connection. We never know where the conversations will go or what emotions will rise to the surface, but we do know that it is our work as carers to give people something to hold that will connect them to the world again and to other people. It also falls to us to listen very deeply to the people we care for to try and understand what emotions they want to convey to us. We don't always succeed. Sometimes the message is just too garbled or we are too tired or stressed to hear the meaning behind the words. But later on, or maybe tomorrow, we will try again, sometimes succeeding in connecting, sometimes failing to connect, but never giving up.

CHET'S STORY

Chet had been an outdoors man all of his life. Now that he was living in a care home he kept to himself, never joining in any social activities or even talking very much. One day we brought in our fishing exercise. We opened up a tackle box filled with fishing paraphernalia: matching pairs of lures (hooks removed and replaced by spinners), a reel, various kinds of plastic bait, different-sized bobbers and matching pairs of laminated fishing-related photos. We use matching work often in our Montessori program because it is a very effective way to focus people on the work. Finding a match is a natural part of our brains' need to look for patterns. Once people find the matching object or matching picture, we discuss what we have matched.

When Chet saw all of the fishing work out on the table in the sitting room of the home, he happily joined us. Chet easily matched the lures and the photos, and then began talking to us about his love of fishing for bluegill fish. We handed him a small rod with a weight on the end of the line. Chet demonstrated to the group his technique for casting and reeling in. His face was alive with happiness and he delighted in talking about the big ones that got away and the various lakes and rivers he fished. From that day on, whenever we came to work in the home where Chet was living, he immediately engaged us in discussions about fishing for bluegill. He never remembered exactly who we were, or our names, but he always remembered that we were the people who brought in the fishing exercise.

This is only one example of the power of finding the right objects to share with people living with dementia. In Chet's case, we had tried for months to engage him and nothing had worked. Bringing in the fishing exercise was the key that unlocked his memories. Even on the days when we didn't bring in the fishing exercise, Chet still joined us and the work we brought in that day. This is the "halo effect." If we are part of a happy occasion or a meaningful moment, then people tend to become more open with us and are often happy to see us, even if they don't remember us or the experiences we've shared.

Exercises and activities

Part of our mission is to find exercises and activities that will be meaningful for men. Of course, many activities are crossovers and attract both men and women. However, after working in many long-term care homes and adult day centers, we realized that there were not enough activities that men found interesting. With this in mind, we developed several activities, such as the fishing exercise. We also created a hub cap polishing exercise (using non-toxic polish). We work with samples of different types of wood, model trains and cars, woodworking exercises, and games about different types of sports. We found small baseball pennants and created a game in which the participants decide which teams are in the National League and which teams are in the American League. The participants place the pennant under a card that reads National League or American League. This game can easily be modified to be used for soccer (football) or many other sports.

Once again, the idea behind creating these types of exercises and activities is to connect with people living with dementia and to give them opportunities to socialize, reminisce, and to share their feelings. We are, at heart, social beings, and we need to be listened to and to feel that we are needed and valued. Sometimes when we see a person with dementia sitting and staring (that thousand-mile stare) it may seem as though there is nothing there. It can feel like the person who once occupied that body is no longer with us. It is our mission to reach that person locked away by dementia. We keep trying until we find the song, the photograph, the poem, the object that clears the fog of dementia and they are with us once again, even if only for a brief moment.

G.K. Chesterton, a well-regarded English poet, writer, and philosopher, wrote this about memory loss in his book, *Orthodoxy*:

> We have all read in scientific books, and, indeed, in all romances, the story of the man who has forgotten his name. This man walks about the streets and can see and appreciate everything; only he cannot remember who he is. Well, every man is that man in the story. Every man has forgotten who he is. One may understand the cosmos, but never the ego; the self is more distant than any star. Thou shalt love the Lord thy God; but thou shalt not know thyself. We are all under the same mental calamity; we have all forgotten our names. We have all forgotten what we really are. All that we call common sense and rationality and practicality and positivism means that for certain dead levels of our life we forget that we have forgotten. All that we call spirit and art and ecstasy only means that for one awful instant we remember that we forgot.[8]

Taking care of the carers

We found this passage of Chesterton's to be particularly meaningful for those of us engaged in the caring professions. We can sometimes find ourselves slipping into the wounded healer role—so exhausted, depleted, and afraid that we don't do what needs to be done to care for ourselves. We don't see how we can manage to be carers and still take care of our own physical, emotional, and spiritual needs. This is the "dead levels of our life," the flat country from where there seems to be no escape. And now, we, the carers are the ones longing for yesterday, longing for a time when life seemed normal and we had the time and energy to do the things that empowered us and gave us joy. That is why it is essential for carers to find a person or group who will listen to their stories and give them comfort, even if just for a few hours.

A wife of a man living in a memory enhancement center called us one day to ask if we thought it would be alright if she took a few days off to take a little vacation. Her voice shook with emotion and we could tell that this phone call was very difficult for her to make. Of course, we encouraged her to take as much time as she felt she needed. We assured her that the staff at the center where her husband lived would look after him. But that wasn't what worried her. What was troubling her was the thought of how angry her husband would be if she left him for a few days. She told us, "I'm afraid my going away isn't worth the anger and grief it will cause him." Again, we reassured her that an important part of her husband's care plan was her own wellbeing, and that she should go, relax, have some fun, and leave the worries and the guilt behind.

If you don't feel comfortable physically leaving the person you care for, you can always build time for yourself into your daily routine. Try to take time to chat with friends, have a long bath, read a favorite book, or watch a film or TV show, spend an hour at a spa, go for a swim, or work in the garden. Some of you are probably thinking, "Are they out of their minds? How am I going to find time to do these things? Not possible!" We know how difficult it can be to take just an hour or two away from your caregiving duties. But as you probably already know, taking time to recharge is vital for your health and the wellbeing of the person you care for. Please don't be shy or hesitant to engage friends and family to take over for you for an hour, half a day, or all day, so that you can give yourself the time you need to find yourself again, to reconnect with your own spirit, to refresh your relationship with you, to remember your own name, and to honor who you are, deep in your soul. The person with dementia is not the only one who needs to be deeply listened to; you also need that. Your needs, your fears, your hopes need to be heard, too. Find someone who will give to you what you give to others: someone who will take the time to listen and to really hear what you are saying.

I AM
SPEAKING

Do you understand me? Do you feel what I am feeling? Do I have your undivided attention? Are you listening to me?

Every day is a journey, and the journey itself is home. (Matsuo Basho)

Chapter Four

The Storied Memory

Have you ever seen an MRI of the brain that was taken when a person is reading? These fMRIs (functional Magnetic Resonance Imaging) show that when we read, our brains light up like a Christmas tree. Reading is a global brain experience. We have found that *reading is a tool that can be very effective in helping us reach people living with dementia.* We encourage carers and family members to provide lots of opportunity for reading. If a person no longer has the capability to read themselves, then we encourage their friends and carers in long-term care homes or adult day centers to read aloud to them. At home, family members, especially children, can read aloud to their elders. We suggest that after reading a page or two, stop and engage the person listening in a discussion. This helps the listener keep track of the story or article, and makes the reading experience more engaging. We also encourage staff to ask people who can still read to take the role of official reader. We have seen that giving a person with dementia a specific role within a community leads to feelings of confidence and wellbeing.

GEORGIA DEE'S STORY

Georgia Dee was a tough woman with advanced Alzheimer's living in a rural long-term care setting. Georgia Dee could be very aggressive toward the other residents and staff, often rolling over toes in her wheelchair, shoving people she perceived were in her path, or pinching people on the backside. Georgia Dee had worked as a truck driver and farmer and raised a large family. She lived a hardscrabble life and had little patience for other people.

One day, quite by accident, we realized that Georgia Dee could read. She was turning over the pieces of a wooden puzzle, reading aloud where the puzzle was manufactured. We handed Georgia Dee a binder with a short story we had written. It was printed in a large font (18+ point) and was a story of an Indiana farmer (see Pat's story later). Georgia Dee read the story to herself and then she spontaneously began reading the story aloud. As she read, several residents gathered around her. Georgia Dee glanced up at her audience, sat up straighter in her wheelchair, and began reading in a louder, more dramatic voice. When she finished reading the story, we asked her and the group some open-ended questions such as,

"Why do you think the farmer named his cow Old Jewell?"

These types of questions are meant to encourage conversation and connection; there are no right or wrong answers. Conversation is the end goal of the reading exercises we create. It is another strategy to help people connect to others and to their own memories.

Our elder reading program is two-pronged: it is designed to keep people reading for as long as possible as well as promoting listening to others reading aloud and creating conversations about these readings. Our elder reading program centers around the stories we gather from people who are living with dementia—we find that elders tend to empathize deeply with stories relating to their peers and their own generation.

Recording stories

As mentioned in Chapter Three, we encourage people to share their stories by giving them something meaningful to hold in their hands. This is our way of priming the pump and sparking memories and conversations. We never know what stories these objects will elicit and are often very surprised by what we hear. We write down these stories and then reproduce them in large print, printing several copies, and placing each copy in its own binder with a photo of the main subject (a train, a church, a farm, etc.). We enhance the narratives by printing up photos to accompany the stories. We have also brought in music that fits with the story and play it after we read. Or we might bring in objects that help illustrate something that happened in the story. We once reproduced a story that an elder told us about his first ride on a steam train. We brought in a CD of train songs and set up a toy steam train on a table in the living room of the memory clinic.

We make ten copies of each story. We do this to facilitate elders reading aloud to each other in an elder reading circle. In these circles, each person reads one page and then the next page is read by someone else. We encourage conversations about these stories and find that the stories told by older people and read aloud by older people often strike a chord that other types of stories don't. Here is an example of a story given to us by a retired pastor who was living with Parkinson's dementia:

THE PASTOR'S STORY

It was just after the war (Second World War) where I'd served as a sailor on a submarine. I went to college on the G.I. Bill [Servicemen's Readjustment Act of 1944] but had no idea what I wanted to study. My shoelace came untied one day while I was walking through the college campus and I stopped to tie it. When I looked up I saw that I was in front of the School of Divinity and thought to myself, why not? I eventually became an ordained minister and was assigned to be the pastor in a small church in upstate New York. I was newly married and this was my first church as an ordained minister.

I visited all the homes in the town, inviting people to come to my church. In one of the houses I visited, I met a young woman who had a small child, a little girl. When I extended the invitation to join us at next Sunday's church service, the young mother shook her head no, and told me that she couldn't come because she wasn't married and had no idea where her child's father was. She believed that the congregation would shun her and her little daughter. I convinced her that she would be very welcome in our church and she reluctantly agreed to join us.

Before the church service that Sunday morning, I asked all the men in my congregation to join me in the church for a short meeting. As the men looked up at me on the altar, I took off my robe, rolled up my shirt sleeves, and told the men that I had invited this young woman who had a child but was not married to come to the service that morning. I told the men that if any of them had a problem with her attending our church they should meet me out back and we would duke it out! The men grumbled but none of them took me up on the offer to fight. That young woman and her little girl attended church that Sunday and all the other Sundays that I was assigned to that church.

After I retired, my wife and I drove back to that first church to look around and reminisce about how we began our lives together there. My wife found the church bulletin from a recent Sunday service and, to our amazement, we saw that the church organist was the little girl who had come to church with her unmarried mother. Now she was an older woman herself, and still a member of that church!

The end.

We've shared this story with people who are of different faiths or people who ascribe to no religious beliefs. We've had people read this story aloud together in many different regions of the US. No matter what group reads the story, it always leads to lively discussions. That is the reason we collect and share these stories from our elders. They speak to the customs and mores of times past. The people who participate in our elder reading circles recognize their fellow elder stories and relate to them profoundly. We feel honored to collect and share these stories. We cannot stress enough the importance of elders reading stories told by people of their own generation. Here is another story we share with the elders we work with. It was told to us by two women who immigrated to the US from Scandinavia, Jenny and Esther. We were working on the Montessori flag exercise—small flags from all over the world are placed in a wooden stand with holes in it. When they found the flag from Norway, Jenny began to reminisce about leaving her homeland. She began the story with her leaving Norway when she was 14:

JENNY'S STORY

I remember seeing the fields of poppies in Norway when the ship pulled away from the shore. I had to start school in the US in first grade. I was 14 years old so it was very hard for me to fit into the little desks and all the small children laughed at me. After a few months, when my English was pretty good, I was allowed to move into sixth grade class. I attended school in America until I was 16 and got married. I didn't get my high school diploma then, but later I took that test and they gave me a diploma. I was proud of that.

I married a man who was from Norway too. He was older than me and had his own bakery. I worked for him for some time and then he said he thought we would make good partners. People in those days didn't talk about love or things like you see in the movies. We found someone who seemed nice and if we thought we would make a good team, then we got married. I didn't love him at first but I needed him and he needed me. So maybe later on we loved each other. I don't know. I only know we were a good team and made a go of that bakery. It was my job every morning to go down to the shop (we lived above the bakery) at three in the morning to get the ovens started so it would be hot for him when he came downstairs.

Esther interrupted her friend here. She elbowed Jenny in the side and said,

"I bet you kept it hot for him!"

The two ladies fell into peals of laughter at this wry remark. Esther then continued with her story.

ESTHER'S STORY

My family was like those books, *Little House on the Prairie*. We lived in a sod house in Montana. I loved that sod house. It was cool in the summer and warm in the winter. Our family helped start the first church and the first school in that area. We brought a little harmonium with us in the covered wagon so I could keep up my music. I remember the wild roses that grew alongside the banks of the creek. Sometimes, I can still smell those roses!

It should be noted that these stories are not especially dramatic. They often do not address major historical events or major life events. Instead, they are like snapshots, moments in time from a long life. But the stories do speak of the courage, determination, and unique experiences that shape one's life.

When we began this work, we tried many different strategies and techniques to find inroads to the people we were trying to reach. When we placed something of meaning in a person's hand and had that breakthrough moment, we were often amazed by the memories and the stories the objects inspired. It was as though we were given gifts by these older people: life lessons, simple stories that held within them beautiful moments of courage, love, joy, and sometimes, sadness. We feel fortunate that we are able to collect and share the stories we hear. It has always been our goal to discover new ways to reach elders and to assist carers as they strive to find the best ways to connect with the people they care for. However, we didn't know that we would be the beneficiaries of so much wisdom and humor. These stories have touched our lives and the lives of the people who participate in our elder reading circles and their caregivers.

Games and exercises

Along with story reading, we've developed *several games and exercises* as part of our elder reading program, all of which are designed to strengthen and maintain the reading abilities of people living with dementia. One very popular game is *Name that Tune*. This game provides reading practice for the participants, as well as helping to ground them in the moment. The person who is guiding the game has cards with the first part of song titles printed on them (we always use large print when creating cards for participants). The people who are playing the game hold the cards with the last word of the song title. We've found that the people participating always begin to the sing the songs they've named. They may also begin to share memories of songs they sang or songs that were popular when they were young.

Another game we've developed that is quite similar to *Name that Tune* is *Finish the Phrase.* This is a game based on proverbs commonly used in conversation such as, "A stitch in time saves...?"

The cards we create for these word-finding games are printed in 72 point (one inch) using a sans serif font, such as Arial or **Helvetica**. These types of fonts are easier to read because they are simple and straightforward. We also laminate the cards to increase their longevity and to ease cleaning of the cards between uses. As it is essential to give people living with dementia something concrete to hold in their hands, people playing these or other games are able to focus more actively when they have cards to hold in their hands. Asking them to come up with answers out of thin air is difficult and frustrating; the simple act of creating cards for them to hold eliminates many of these difficulties.

These sorts of games are excellent for helping make connections when people come to visit their friends or loved ones living in an intentional community. These games can be led by staff members, family members, or by elders who are functioning at a fairly high level. Families can also use these games at home with elders. We have found these types of word-finding games to be an excellent tool to help different generations connect with each other. Again, the goal of these exercises is to give elders opportunities to practice their remaining reading skills, to promote socialization and reminiscence, and to give staff, family, and friends the tools to connect with people living with dementia.

Activities such as holding cards and reading are based in procedural memory (muscle memory). Because the procedural memory system tends to be more intact throughout the course of dementia, we try to incorporate it into all of the exercises that we create. Giving people cards to hold engages their hands and helps them focus on the current activity. Reading itself is part of the procedural memory system. When we read, our eyes move back and forth, engaging the eye muscles. Of course, some people living with dementia do lose their ability to read. That is why we encourage reading aloud and why we created the elder reading circle and reading games as activities for those who can still read as well as for those who can no longer read but who can participate by listening.

There is another reading game we play that engages the procedural memory system and also stimulates the mind. It is a game created by Dr. Montessori called *Category Sort*. The game is based on the fact that people store different categories in different parts of the brain. For example, the idea of a puppy is stored in one part of the brain while the idea of a hammer is stored in a different part of the brain. We build on this knowledge of the brain to create exercises that can stimulate and challenge the mind. It may initially seem odd to consider challenging someone who is already struggling with dementia. However, if the challenge is structured to the individual and is fun and engaging, we've found that people living with dementia can enjoy a challenge.

In *Category Sort* games, we find two groups of objects that are the opposite of each other. So, if one group is "things that are living," the opposite group would be "things that are not living." Here is a sample of this game. We create cards, 6 x 8 inches, with large print so that people have something to hold in their hands and can practice their reading skills:

LIVING	NOT LIVING
• SUN	• WIND
• SPIDER	• WOOL
• FROG	• WINDMILL
• WORM	• FIRE
• MOUSE	• FIRE TRUCK
• DAFFODIL	• LEATHER
• FISH	• CLOUD
• ROSE	• COTTON

Participants hold a card printed with one of the words listed above. They place the card under the "Living" category or under the "Not living" category. There is no right or wrong answer in these exercises. We once had a farmer argue passionately that a tractor is a living thing. He told the group that he and his old girl (his tractor) had worked together in the fields for years and years and that she was as

fe. These exercises are designed
also to stimulate conversations

Sort exercises could be created
:

ol box/Objects found in a purse.

ter/Clothes worn in summer.

y/Foods that taste sweet.

y creating cards using large print
as a tool box filled with plastic
akeup, a wallet, etc.

se we created (which has become a big hit with elders in many different parts of the country and in all kinds of settings) is a humor-based game. We print up a series of jokes, one joke per card. On one side of the card is the set-up for the joke. The person then flips the card over to read the punch line. For example, someone holding a card reads, "What nationality is Santa Claus?" then flips the card over and reads the punch line, "North Polish!" Full disclosure, some of these jokes are very corny, as in, they're real groaners, like "What did the dog eat for breakfast?"…"Barkin' and eggs." But others bring real belly laughs. Here is a joke that has proven to be the favorite for all the groups we've worked with:

Set-up:

> What did the bra say to the top hat?

Flip the card over and the punch line reads:

You go on ahead. I'll give these two
A LIFT!

An interesting phenomenon occurred when we started using joke cards in our work. We would give each participant half a dozen jokes to read aloud. A person would begin to read the jokes and have to be prompted to turn the card over to get to the punch line on the back. By the time the participants got to joke number four or five, they were remembering on their own to flip the card over to read the punch line. We also noticed that many of the participants would get into the rhythm of joke telling. They would pause for just a moment before delivering the punch line. A simple and funny exercise such as reading jokes aloud brings so much joy and laughter to the people living with dementia and their carers. When we're laughing together, our spirits are lifted and we are bound closer together.

Trivia is a word game that is often used in care homes and adult day centers. We've developed our own version of a *Trivia* game that has proven to be very popular and effective in dementia units and memory enhancement centers. We begin each game by choosing one topic. It may be types of flowers or US presidents or old movies, but we always just use one category per game. We might use presidents one day and then favorite films the next day, but the categories are always kept separate. We do this so that the people playing the *Trivia* game will experience less confusion and be more successful.

As we do in other word-finding games, we create cards for people to hold that are printed in very large print (72 point or larger), for ease of reading. Each card has a correct answer printed on it. If, for example, the group is playing *Trivia* about presidents, each participant would get one or two or three cards (depending on the size of the group) printed with the last name of a different president. The person running the *Trivia* game has a book with the questions and answers. They also have a large card with the question written on it and three possible answers, a, b, or c, that they hold up so that the group can read the card as the question is being asked:

Which US president had a beard and wore a stovepipe hat?

a Donald Trump
b Teddy Roosevelt
c Abraham Lincoln

One person in the group will be holding the correct answer card (Abraham Lincoln).

The correct answer for all of our *Trivia* questions is always the third answer, "c." When the group begins playing *Trivia*, some of the people see the pattern right away (that the correct answer is always the third answer). Others may take longer to see the pattern and a few never catch on. There was one woman who was playing our version of *Trivia* and was getting a lot of correct answers. She told the group, "I know the right answers but I don't know how I know them."

She had, in fact, figured out the pattern that the right answer was always the last answer. We designed our *Trivia* game in this manner after observing that, in many traditional *Trivia* games, one or two people in the group would answer all of the questions. We wanted to give everyone a chance to get the correct answer. We also provide cards for people to hold to help them focus on the game. Each *Trivia* game is played using only one category so that the participants are not confused by too many different kinds of questions. And, as we always say, these games are created to promote socialization and to help people with dementia connect once again with their community and with their loved ones.

As with many of the Montessori games and exercises that we create, carers are only limited by their own imaginations. We understand that time and energy levels are major considerations and that is why we suggest activities that are simple to make and that don't take inordinate amounts of time. A family carer can enlist the help of other family members or friends to help in the creation of these games and exercises, and we also encourage family members and friends to participate. These games and exercises can be a bridge to reach and stay connected to people living with dementia. They can also be a lot of fun and lead to some interesting conversations and moments of laughter and joy.

Two reading circle stories

We want to leave you with two more of our elder reading circle stories, which have journeyed to places all over the world. Everyone who reads these stories finds them to be a special chronicling of a time when life was very tough and the people who survived had to be even tougher.

Rebecca was 95 years old when we first met her. She had a wonderful memory for times past but was never sure of who we were or why we came to the long-term care home where she now lived. Knowing this, we would introduce ourselves every time we came to work with her. Rebecca was a well-trained and enthusiastic musician. We knew that if we asked her to play something on the piano, this procedural memory experience (playing the piano) would bring forth stories and memories of her early life in Chicago.

REBECCA'S STORY: THE BEST GIFT

The calendar said it was spring, but winter wasn't quite finished with us yet. This particular Saturday started with a cold rain, and as the temperature continued to drop, the rain turned to sleet. The sidewalks were soon covered with ice. As I climbed the steps to the El train downtown after work, a flower vendor's colorful display caught my eye. It seemed so out of place to see fresh roses in that miserably cold corner. They weren't long stemmed, but they were roses!

Suddenly, I felt a tremendous urge to buy a dozen roses and bring them to my friend, Mae. Mae was a soloist in our choir. I was her accompanist and I admired her tremendously. This was during the depression, so even 25 cents was big money for me. The vendor gave me extra wax paper to protect the roses and I headed for home.

My mom was appalled when I told her of my planned errand to take the roses to Mae. As I gulped down a little of her good dinner, her words to me were, "In this terrible weather?"

After slipping and sliding for blocks, taking a short ride on the Western Avenue streetcar and a longer ride on the Milwaukee Avenue streetcar, plus three more blocks of walking and sliding, I finally reached her address, but no Mae. Her grimly angry mother-in-law told me, "They've moved out!"

After considerable pleading she gave me their new address. Another three-block hike brought me back to

Milwaukee Avenue and the factory-type building where Mae now lived. No front door entrance, no side door entrance. After picking my way through mud and debris, I found a rickety door at the back of the building. Inside was a long, dark stairway. With my heart in my throat, I inched my way up the stairs and knocked on the door.

The door opened and Mae's husband stood in the doorway with their toddler in his arms. His inability to find work had led to the quarrel with his parents and their telling him to leave.

He told me Mae was walking to her mother's home to ask for money for bread and milk for the baby. By now, I was feeling that the roses were totally inappropriate, but her husband's eyes were glistening as he put the flowers in a tall water glass. His voice wasn't quite steady as he told me, "When Mae left to go see her mother, she said, 'I don't think there is one person in this whole world who cares whether we live or die.'"

They both told me afterward of the tears that flowed when Mae returned home to find roses waiting for her. Through the years she often mentioned that little bunch of roses as the best gift she had ever received.

The end.

When we read this story in elder reading circles, we always ask the group this question:

"What color were the roses in Rebecca's story?"

There isn't a right or wrong answer to this question because we never asked Rebecca what color the roses were. Now it's too late to ask her, so we'll just have to guess. What color do you think the roses were?

The second story was told to us by a man living in a rural community. This story is simple, but it has a deep lesson to teach us—that we are all connected, sentient and non-sentient beings, we all belong.

PAT'S STORY: OLD JEWELL

My father-in-law was a dairy farmer. He spent his entire working life on a farm in New England building up a first-class herd of Holsteins. He not only worked at improving the breed of milking cows; he conscientiously cared for them. The barn was always clean. The stalls had fresh straw and the animals were well fed. The cows all had individual names. Dad used their names soothingly as he worked with them, brushing their hides, or doing the milking twice a day. He talked to them constantly whenever he worked around them.

One time when I was spending a few days at the farm with my family, I was awakened in the middle of the night by a loud noise outside the window. Someone or something was crashing around in the garden, bumping over the bean poles, and kicking against the fence. I knew in an instant what was happening. One of the cows had gotten out of the barn and was in the garden. She was now away from the rest of the herd in an unfamiliar place and unable to find her way back. You could hear her thrashing around, panic-stricken in the unfamiliar surroundings. At that time, my father-in-law was getting older and I thought that I would help him by saving him the trouble of having to get up in the middle of the night. I called into his bedroom that I would get the cow and take her back to the barn.

"That's probably old Jewell," he called back. "She's always getting into trouble. You may not be able to handle her!"

In a moment, I was dressed and in the garden. But when I tried to approach the panic-stricken animal, I only frightened her. She began to bellow and thrash around more. When I touched her, she tossed her head and reared off in a different direction. Try as I might, I could not get that cow to go back through the gate and into the barnyard. She did not know me, and my presence added to her confusion.

Suddenly Dad arrived. His walk and manner were slow and deliberate as always. Then his strong baritone voice pierced the night:

"Jewell!" he called.

Immediately, and as if by magic, the old cow stopped her thrashing around and stood still. Even in the darkness, Dad had known which cow it was. She, in turn, had immediately recognized his voice when he called her name. I stood in amazement and watched my father-in-law go up to the large animal, thump her a few love taps, and then walk her through the gate and back to the rest of the herd where she once again was safe.

My father-in-law turned to me and said very simply,

"I know my own and my own know me."

The end.

As stated earlier, we gather these stories from the people we work with and transform them into written stories. We create several copies of each story, reproducing them in at least 18 point or larger, using sans serif fonts and placing each story in a binder. We often have ten copies of one story, each in their own binder. We may illustrate the story with pictures or photographs, or we may bring in objects that add points of interest. When we print the stories, we make sure to have each page end on a complete sentence. This makes it easier when people take turns reading the story: one page per person. The discussions after the story can be led by a staff person, a family member, or one of the people living with dementia who might enjoy guiding the conversation.

Elder reading circles can be created in an intentional community or in a family home. These reading groups provide a wonderful opportunity for intergenerational interactions. Gathering, creating, and sharing these stories from our elders keeps them and their memories alive. Within these stories their wisdom, love, humor, grit, failures, and successes live on. We remember our lives in stories. Sometimes the stories are just a flash of memory, a snapshot in time. At other times, there is an entire narrative, beginning, middle, and end. This is the storied memory. Our stories are how we remember our lives and how we share our lives. We are our stories.

It takes a thousand voices to tell a single story. (Native American proverb)

Chapter Five

Dementia and Creativity

JANIE'S STORY

We sat with Janie as she concentrated with great attention on her painting. Her nose almost touched the paper as she swirled a vivid red color across the middle of the paper with her brush. She talked as she painted, "See, this is where the robbers got into the house. Now, we have to get those children out because those bad men have started a fire."

The house she so carefully created was now filled with red flames. Suddenly she stopped painting, sighed, and leaned back in her chair. She was finished with both the art and the story. Janie looked at us and smiled, very content, very relaxed. We wondered if there was some reason that she painted this painting and told us this story. Had something like this happened in her past? Had someone jeopardized her children? Had she been the victim of a fire or a robbery? We asked her daughter about this when she came to visit later that day. She thought for a moment and then shrugged her shoulders,

"If something like that happened, I never heard of it. I think Mom was making a movie in her head."

Making movies in our heads is what we hope will happen when we set up painting projects. As with all of the exercises and activities we create for our Montessori program, the end goal is communication and reconnection. Many of the people we work with are reluctant to try painting. Most have never painted a picture in their lives. The first thing we have to do when we start a painting class is help participants get over their fears or shyness. Initial resistance is often due to the fact that many older people were exposed to a very regimented and highly critical form of education. Over time, they have become reluctant to try new things, as they are afraid of making a mistake or doing it "wrong." This is what we hear when we work with elders, that they would like to try something but they're sure they'll get it wrong. A great joy of our work is helping people gather up the courage to try something new and watching them discover that they truly enjoy it.

As Sir Ken Robinson, author and educator, so wisely wrote, "We are all born with extraordinary powers of imagination, intelligence, feeling, intuition, spirituality, and of physical and sensory awareness."[9] Being totally present with the people with whom we are working is one of the true joys of connecting to people living with dementia.

We were working in a long-term care home, setting up several table easels, paints, and brushes when a dairy farmer approached us.

"I can show you how to milk a cow but you ain't never gonna get me to paint no picture!" We didn't argue with him but invited him to stay and watch the painting class.

After watching several people around him painting away, the farmer picked up a paint brush and begin to dab some color on the paper. In a few minutes, he was busy filling the entire page with dots and dots of color. When he finished with his painting, he grinned at us and said, "Now don't expect me to cut off my ear! It ain't no Whistler's *Mother*."

He may have had his artists confused, but the dairy farmer was very pleased with his first painting and hung it with pride in his bedroom.

When we set up a painting program in a long-term care home, memory unit, or adult day center, we adhere to the Montessori principle of isolating the difficulty and breaking the exercise down to its most basic steps. We keep it very elemental so that we don't overwhelm the participants. We have found that if we make the painting project simple, it is easier for people with dementia to give it a try. With this in mind, we only bring in the three primary colors, red, yellow, and blue. Each person has three small containers, and each container holds either the color red, yellow, or blue, along with a paint brush. There is a small bowl that holds water to clean the brushes. The paints we use are non-toxic and washable. We use small table easels, or if these aren't available, we use squares of compressed wood (14 x 14 inches) as easels. We use compressed wood because it is smooth and won't hurt the participants' hands or rip the paper. The paper we use is 8 x 12 inches. We find that smaller paper is less intimidating. When we use the compressed wood squares as easels, we tape the paper to the squares using masking tape. Some of the elders like to help us tape the paper to the squares. We discovered that when the participants help set up the painting project, they are more apt to join in the painting.

Understanding that many people living with dementia struggle with failure to initiate, we find that it is helpful to sit quietly beside them while they decide if they can begin the project. Sometimes, we pick up a paint brush and just put a dot or two of color on the paper. Often, that is enough to encourage someone to try to paint. We don't suggest what they should paint or ask them to copy another painting. We encourage the participants to create whatever they wish. This can be difficult for people who struggle with the concept of making something out of nothing (moving from the abstract to the concrete). The idea of filling up a blank piece of paper can be intimidating and challenging, especially if a person has never even held a paint brush. Early on, we found that group painting was the most successful approach for creating art. Seeing others making all sorts of different paintings gives people a bit of courage and the motivation to try painting themselves.

The paintings we've seen elders create differ wildly. Some people fill up the paper with color. Someone else may put one solitary dot on the page and be done. One person we worked with would only paint the masking tape that held the paper; he would never paint on the paper itself. Others try representational painting, creating a house or a farm field or flowers. We never correct someone's effort or guess what they were trying to paint. In the Montessori Method, it is the process that matters, not the product. People create whatever they want to create. We don't pass judgment on it or try and decipher it. It is the participants' joy in creativity that we are seeking. There is such a sense of confidence and wellbeing that comes over a person when they complete their own creation. These feelings may last only a few minutes, but it is worth everything to see the expression of satisfaction on the artist's face. The poet, Dylan Thomas, wrote beautifully about this concept of free-form painting in his poem, "A Child's Christmas in Wales":

> ... And a painting book in which I could make the grass, the trees, the sea and the animals any color I please, and

still the dazzling sky-blue sheep are grazing in the red field under the rainbow-billed and pea-green birds.

By Dylan Thomas, from A Child's Christmas in Wales, *copyright © 1954 by New Directions Publishing Corp. Reprinted by permission of New Directions Publishing Corp.*

Dylan Thomas understood so very well the idea that it doesn't matter what we create as long as we are allowed to bring forth what we feel, what we see, and what we want to share.

This opportunity to share emotions and ideas is central to our art program. Many people living with dementia lose the ability to communicate through language, either written language or spoken language. At the same time that they lose the ability to talk about their emotions, they are often barraged with feelings of fear, anxiety, and frustration. We have found that painting is an effective way to give people a chance to express themselves again. Painting can be a tremendous relief for people who have no other way to cope with their fears and worries.

We have also observed in these painting groups that people often bond while creating art. They talk with each other about what they're doing, encouraging each other, and enjoying one another's work. And, of course, there is the added bonus of sharing artwork within the intentional community or with families. We encourage the staff or family members to frame the work and display it for other people to enjoy. Oftentimes, the artists won't remember that the painting is their work, but somewhere, deep inside, there remains that spark of living in the moment that comes from creating art.

Another important part of our art program is bringing in paintings and small sculptures to share with elders. We place the different paintings on an easel, one at a time, and discuss the painting with the group. Again, we start conversations with open-ended questions:

Why do you think the woman in this painting is smiling?

How do you think the man in the boat is feeling?

Libraries are an excellent resource for borrowing paintings or small sculptures. Sculptures are especially meaningful for people who have limited sight. They can feel the sculptures and join in a discussion about art. We've had some amazing conversations about these works of art. In Renoir's painting, *Dance at Bougival*, the central figures are a couple dancing. As they dance, the man is looking intently at the woman but she is looking down and away from him. One of the elders who was studying this painting said to us, "He's crazy about her but she doesn't really like him, does she?"

It was an astute observation and led to a lively conversation in the group about relationships between men and women, dances they attended, and people they had dated when they were young.

MAXINE'S STORY

We were working in a long-term care home and brought in several paintings to show the residents. We came to this home once a week to work with people who had dementia. One of the people we worked with, Maxine, had never spoken a word. Everyone assumed that she was mute. The group was studying Winslow Homer's painting, *The Gulf Stream*, of a lone man, his foot shackled to a small sailing boat as an ocean storm rages about him and sharks circle the boat. Maxine went up to the painting and peered closely at it.

Then she turned to the group and announced, "He seems very nonchalant, doesn't he?"

We all sat there for a moment, absolutely shocked that Maxine had spoken and that she came out with such a profound observation. Maxine went on speaking. She told us that she and her husband used to go to the local art museum all the time and it was one of her favorite things to do. After that breakthrough moment, Maxine continued to talk to us and to the people where she lived. There was something in Homer's painting that spoke deeply to Maxine and unlocked her ability to speak. It was a very moving moment for us. This is what we've come to understand about our work in the field of dementia: you never know what experience will reach a person living with dementia and that's why we have to keep trying. That's why we never give up on anyone.

Marilyn Raichle's mother, Jean, was diagnosed with Alzheimer's when she was in her late eighties. She faced this diagnosis with courage and grace, telling her family to "walk away" when the time comes. "I won't remember you anyway." Jean's daughter, Marilyn, did not walk away but instead, chose to walk this Alzheimer's journey with her mother. One of the saving graces of this journey was Jean's growing interest in painting. She had never painted in her life, but when presented with the opportunity to join the painting classes going on in the long-term care home where Jean lived, she decided to give painting a try and never looked back. Creating art became a large part of Jean's life and, to her great surprise, art created by people living with dementia became a large part of Marilyn's life, too. Here is their story as told by Marilyn:

MARILYN'S STORY

Anne Basting, an American gerontologist specializing in applied arts in long-term care and dementia, says, "While access to language may falter, the imagination can soar."

At the age of 89, living with mid-stage Alzheimer's, my mother Jean surprised us all and began to paint. She had warned us, "When my time comes, walk away. I won't remember you anyway." And we believed her. But her paintings were filled with life and wit, confounding everything I thought I knew about Alzheimer's. I began to share her art with friends and family and the reaction was always the same—surprise, delight, and gratitude to experience a story about Alzheimer's that was filled with joy and hope. When I told her how much people enjoyed her art, she laughed in disbelief, and said, "They're crazy!" When pressed, she would say, "I must have gotten this from your father's side of the family."

Inspired by Mom, our first exhibition, *The Artist Within*, featured 51 exhilarating paintings by 41 vibrant persons, aged 60 to 101, all living with dementia. Delightful, surprising, and inspiring, they effortlessly told a story—they are *still here*, living with dignity, creativity, and joy.

The creative arts have a profound ability to enrich the lives of persons living with memory loss and dementia. In the joy and intensity of creation, relationships are built and strengthened, anxiety and depression eased, and a sense of mastery or control over their environment is developed. This was certainly true for Mom, and for all of us, the impact of the arts is equally important. Art effortlessly connects us, overcoming stigma, inspiring awareness, expanding knowledge and engagement. These exhilarating paintings invite us to celebrate the creativity and imagination of persons living well with dementia and to strengthen our shared resolve to build a dementia-friendly community. Our new exhibit will display 50 paintings created by seven vibrant persons living with dementia, each sharing a unique view of the world. We will meet them as creative and valuable members of our community.

Although Marilyn's mother is no longer living, her legacy, the love of painting and creating art lives on in her daughter's work with people living with dementia. These paintings not only bring joy to the people who create them; they also uplift all who see them—family members, friends, and the public at large who view the exhibitions that Marilyn sponsors. These are gifts that keep on giving, reminding us all that, as Marilyn so beautifully writes, "They are *still here*, living with dignity, creativity, and joy."

Billie was a person we met in a memory enhancement center who demonstrates Marilyn's thesis, that giving people with dementia the opportunity to create art can lead to surprising outcomes. Billie had painted most of her life, decorating china dishes and china dolls. It was her hobby and her great love. The room she occupied at the center held an armoire filled with the dishes and china dolls she had painted.

Even though she had so much experience painting, Billie was still hesitant to join the art class. She was diagnosed with Parkinson's and dementia, and told us that she didn't think she could hold a paint brush anymore because her hands shook so badly. Adhering to the Montessori principle of "invite, never insist," we didn't push Billie. She would often join the painting group as an observer, giving pointers to the people painting, and sometimes offering ideas for their creations.

BILLIE'S STORY

One day, Billie sat down at the painting table and picked up a paint brush. She held her right arm steady by gripping her forearm firmly with her left hand. We watched Billie working on a still life of a single, red rose. She created shadows and depths in different shades of red, while the leaves of the rose trailed away, curling and turning with patches of brown and pink and shadings of green. As we watched Billie layering paint, rubbing off the excess with her thumb, the flower, leaves, and vines became luminous under her touch. We told Billie that we would have this glorious rose painting framed for her.

When we met Billie again a few days later, we handed her the painting, matted and framed, the rose looking even more vibrant under the glass. Billie looked at us blankly, not remembering us, not remembering her painting. She shook her head and told us that this was not her work. She insisted that she couldn't paint anymore, that her hands shook too violently for her to hold a paint brush. Relentlessly, Billie's Parkinson's disease was destroying both her mind and her body, but within this destruction there lived the artist, the creator.

Billie sat down at the painting table and stared at the blank paper on the easel. She looked intently at the paint brush resting by the paint pots. With a shaking hand, she smoothed the paper and began drawing on the white emptiness with her index finger. She took a deep breath and then picked up the paint brush, grabbed her right forearm with her left hand, and began to paint. This time an entire garden of flowers jumped to life under her shaking hand. Watching Billie's courageous brush strokes, we were reminded of Ernest Hemingway's words:

> The world breaks everyone, and afterward many are strong at the broken places.

Chapter Six

Drum Circles

GARY'S STORY

We were holding a drum circle in the living room of a memory enhancement center. There were 20 people sitting in a large circle. Some of the participants were holding a frame drum in one hand and a beater in the other hand. Frame drums are thin, lightweight drums with narrow wooden rims. They vary in size, from two feet in circumference to very small drums that are only six inches across. The beaters are small wooden sticks with foam wrapped in leather on the top. The beaters create a sound that resonates but is not loud. Two men and a woman were sitting in front of a large gathering drum with beaters in their hands. Everyone was watching the facilitator in the center of the circle. On this day, the facilitator was one of the residents of the memory center. She guided the group in simple rhythms, ma-ma, da-da. When she raised her arms, the drummers played louder. When she lowered her hands, the drumming grew very quiet. She suddenly made a slashing movement and the group stopped together, instantly. The players then laughed and clapped for their conductor and for themselves.

Gary, a man in his fifties who had been diagnosed with young onset dementia, sat quietly in a corner of the room, observing the drum circle. He sat absolutely still with no expression on his face. When the drumming stopped, the room was suddenly filled with a clicking sound. It was Gary. He was holding a small plastic drinking cup in his hand and clicking ma-ma, da-da. The room grew silent as everyone turned to watch Gary and his plastic cup. He clicked quickly, ma-ma, da-da, and then he clicked slowly, imitating the rhythms he heard the drum circle creating. Tom picked up another plastic cup and answered Gary's rhythm. Gary clicked his plastic cup and stopped, waiting for Tom to answer him. They performed together, Gary initiating the rhythm pattern with his clicking cup and Tom answering him with his cup. When Gary finally tired and put the cup in his lap, the room burst into applause. Gary ducked his head but we saw a glimpse of the small smile that, for an instant, lit up his face. Gary always refused to join the drum circle and he never repeated the plastic cup performance, but in those few fleeting moments that day, Gary was with us. He was very much alive in the moment and it brought him, and all of us, real joy.

In every society, in every culture throughout the world and throughout history, people have gathered in circles. The idea of a circle is associated with important meetings and important discussions. The Knights of the Round Table are a legendary example of an egalitarian meeting of equals to discuss present tactics and future plans. Circle meetings can also signal a more intimate, casual meeting among friends and family.

When we meet in a circle, there is no head, no authority figure. We are all equals in a circle, we face one another and can see other people's reactions. Just sitting in a circle with other people can be a bonding experience. We encourage staff members and administration to use circle meetings to communicate ideas and concerns with each other.

These circle meetings are safe places where people can express their thoughts and emotions without fear of judgment.

We first used the circle formation when establishing our elder reading circles. This was so successful that we began to look for other activities we could present while sitting in a circle. We had attended drum circles with Tom Gill, a well-known and highly respected drum circle leader. Mr. Gill has led drum circles for corporations, schools, and with elders in long-term care homes. This is Tom Gill's introduction to his drum circle program, Rhythm Adventures:[10]

One touch of a drum can fill the air with a resonant *BOOM* or tease the ear with a subdued *whompf*. And then something magical happens: people respond, young and old, playful and serious, curious and nonchalant—all are drawn to the call of the drum beat. We are, after all, rhythmical beings. Our beating heart and our daily habits are all based on cycles. For thousands of years, people have used drums to communicate and to celebrate the rhythms in their lives. All who participate in the practice help to keep the tradition alive.

When I got my first drum, I realized its potential to establish and maintain community togetherness, whether it was within a single family, a neighborhood, or within any group that shares a connection. After years of drumming with various populations, I discovered the joy of sharing the experience with elders in adult day centers and long-term care centers. I was overjoyed when the experience seemed be just what they were looking for!

Many activities for elders involve everyone sitting in rows, facing in the same direction as they watch the action. A circle setting allows everyone to be on equal terms and easily able to interact. People can see, acknowledge, and ultimately open up to one another.

The room set-up is important. Instruments placed in the center of a circle help create a visual focus as people arrive. Seeing familiar (or new) instruments creates a feeling of excitement... The number of participants can vary according to available space, their physical abilities, number of staff present to assist, and the comfort level of the facilitator. Chairs can be mixed with wheelchairs to create a space that meets the needs of the population. Leave room between chairs so people can easily move around to assist in handing out instruments or giving hand-over-hand help to those who need it.

Often older people will tell us that they can't play drums because they don't have any rhythm. We tell them, "If you have a heartbeat, you have rhythm." The frame drums we use in drum circles are lightweight and easy for older people to hold. The beaters we use protect their hands and create a solid, resonant sound without hurting older, more sensitive hands. As well as the lightweight frame drums, we also use Djembe, which are tall, standing, African drums. When available, the gathering drum, a very large drum that stands on its own, is wonderful for drum circles. Two, three, or even four people can play the gathering drum together. We often invite reluctant drummers to join more experienced drummers at the gathering drum.

We begin our drum circles by going around the group and greeting everyone, thanking them for joining us. When the drummers are seated comfortably with their instruments, we invite them to explore the drums, listening to the sounds of the drum and experimenting with beating the drum on the outer edges and right in the middle. The sound of the drum changes as one moves out and in from the center, with the deeper sounds near the middle of the drum head and the higher notes being found toward the outer edge of the drum.

Once people seem comfortable with the drums, the facilitator begins with a simple rhythm. This can be a slow two-beat rhythm that imitates the sound of our own heart when we are resting: da-dum, da-dum, da-dum. We demonstrate the signal for beginning (arms raised) and the signal for stopping (a slashing movement with the hand). Tom Gill likes to start his drum circles by saying, "One-two-ready-play!" He stops the circle by holding up his hand and counting on his fingers, "1-2-3-4-STOP!"[11]

Whatever manner you choose to begin and end the rhythm pattern, as long as you do it the same way consistently, you will find that the group quickly grasps the message you're sending them. We raise our arm high for the drums to play louder and take our hand down low to signal playing quietly. Different facilitators have different ways of instructing the drum circle to play fast or slow.

We find that whatever signals the facilitator chooses to communicate with the drum circle, somehow everyone in the group understands when to start, stop, play quickly, slowly, loudly, softly, and so on. Moreover, the drum circle almost invariably stops together, on a dime. We've observed this phenomenon over and over and have never yet figured out how it happens, how these groups begin to play as one almost instantaneously. Perhaps this happens because we are rhythmic creatures. We hear our mother's heartbeat in the womb, we live with the constant beat of our own hearts. There is a pace at which we walk, at which we move, at which we speak. Drum circles give us the opportunity to share with others the rhythm that lives within us all.

Once the participants in the drum circle are able to play the very simple heartbeat rhythm together, we then move on to four-beat patterns, the ma-ma, da-da rhythm. This simple four beat can be played on a higher note on the drum (near the edge of the drum head) or a lower note (near the center of the drum head). It can be played fast or slow, loudly or softly. Once the group is comfortable with the ma-ma, da-da pattern, the larger group can be divided into two smaller groups, with one group playing only the ma-ma part of the beat and the other half of the group playing only the da-da part of the beat. This is the beginning lesson in the drumming tradition of *call and response*.

Call and response

Call and response is an exercise in which the facilitator of the drum group plays a rhythm pattern and then the drum circle plays the rhythm (the return) back to the facilitator. When the group is comfortable with call and response, any member of the drum circle can create a call that the group will answer. Or the facilitator may have half of the group create a call and the other half of the drum circle will answer the call.

Call and response can be used with any number of beats. It is quite wonderful to see how quickly and easily a drum circle understands and can master call-and-response drumming. As long as the call is simple, the drum circle can almost always respond quite easily.

Tom Gill writes that one of the most useful rhythms to try with drum circles is the following: Mis-sis-sip-pi-Hot (rest) Dog (rest). Each syllable is one beat on the drum. Gill notes that the rest between "Hot" and "Dog" helps bring the group together.[12] Another rhythm pattern that Gill recommends is the 1-2, 1-2-3 or 1-2, cha-cha-cha beat. He states that, "Groups of beats with a slight pause between feel natural and fun to play."[13]

Another simple call-and-response rhythm involves having each person play their own name. Each syllable of a name is a beat on the drum. A drummer named Gloria would play Glor-i-a and the group would respond in kind. Tom also writes that it may take a person a few times acting as the caller before they feel comfortable in this role. As long as the rhythm patterns are kept simple, everyone in the group can be a successful caller and a successful responder.

Extra help

The following are several methods Gill uses to assist people who may need extra help joining a drum circle:

- *Hand over hand*: Gently grasp the hand and mallet of the player to assist him or her in playing a rhythm. You shouldn't force your interpretation of a rhythm; rather, help guide the person. Know if and when it's time to let go so they can react in their own way.

- *Side by side*: Play alongside someone to provide them with a close-up model of how to play an instrument. They can follow along more easily, plus they can feel the enjoyment and support of playing with you as a part of a team.

- *Mirroring*: Crouch down in front of the person and play on their instrument with them so they can mimic your motions. Getting down to their level is important, as standing in front of them will feel like you are towering over them.

- *Verbal and non-verbal encouragement*: Encouragement keeps people engaged and offers the feeling that they are special in that moment. Sometimes all that is needed is to hold the instrument for them. A frame drum held by a helper creates a bond between player and holder.

Other benefits of drumming

Other benefits of drumming, according to Gill, are that the drums can express a person's emotions when words cannot. As with other art forms, drumming can be helpful for people who may have lost the ability to speak or are unable to put their emotions into words. If someone is feeling frustrated and angry, they may find that hitting a drum creates a form of relief from their frustrations and anger. Or, if someone is feeling lonely and sad, being part of a drum circle can help them bond with their peers. There is an intimacy that happens when we play together in a drum circle. There is a tight-knit feeling that grows between people when they are playing the same rhythms together. When we drum together, we come together as one. People who are very shy begin to make eye contact. Others who were reluctant to play the drums are now banging away with alacrity. Drum circles give us the opportunity to listen to each other in an entirely new way. Listening to one another and playing together leads to very real bonding within the group.

Other positive outcomes of drum circles for people living with dementia include an increase in energy levels as well as better focus after participation. There have been several studies on the positive outcomes that drumming may have on people's gait and their ability to walk. One study states that:

Acoustic rhythms are frequently used in gait rehabilitation, with positive instantaneous and prolonged transfer effects on various gait characteristics. The gait modifying ability of acoustic rhythms depends on how well gait is tied to the beat, which can be assessed with measures of relative time of auditory-motor coordination.[14]

JACK'S STORY

We have witnessed this improvement in gait and mobility ourselves. One afternoon, after a lively drum circle that lasted almost an hour, one of the participants (who was diagnosed with Parkinson's disease), Jack, held out his hands and showed us that they were no longer shaking. Jack then began to slowly rise from his chair. One of the staff quickly came to his side, his walker at the ready. The older man waved away the aide and the walker, and slowly began walking by himself across the room, the aide walking close beside him. The look of absolute triumph on this man's face was one we will never forget. The drum circle gave Jack a few moments when he could move and walk again without stiffness or involuntary shaking. And it made him and everyone who watched him that day very happy.

MARGARET'S STORY

There have been a number of remarkable moments that we have observed in drum circles. We were working in an adult day center when one of the clients of the center stormed up to us. She demanded,

"What is all this racket?"

We explained that we were holding a drum circle and invited her to join us.

Margaret raised an eyebrow and stated coldly,

"How can I be part of a group that doesn't even understand triplets? All I hear you playing are two and four beats. And you're not playing those very well!"

We asked the irate woman if she could spare a moment and explain to the group the concept of triplets. Margaret hesitated for a moment and then shrugged her shoulders.

"Oh, alright. Just for a minute."

She stood in the middle of the group and clapped her hands sharply, saying the word "choc-o-late," each syllable accompanied by a clap. Margaret repeated the triple beat, choc-o-late, several times and then invited the drummers to join her in playing a triplet. The group dutifully said "choc-o-late" and played the triplet beat. After a few tries, the drum circle was successfully playing triplets together. Margaret suddenly stopped the group and began singing the chorus of an old song, "On Moonlight Bay." The group quickly joined her, most of them remembering this favorite tune:

We were sailing along
On Moonlight Bay.
We could hear the voices ringing;
They seemed to say,
You have stolen my heart
Now don't go 'way!
As we sang love's old sweet song
On Moonlight Bay.

Margaret began the song again, but this time after singing two lines she clapped out the rhythm for two sets of triplets: choc-o-late, choc-o-late. The drum group soon picked up the pattern and all of a sudden everyone was singing "On Moonlight Bay" and adding the double triplets after every other line. It sounded amazing! When the song finished, the drum circle spontaneously broke into applause and the once irate facilitator smiled and gave a little bow. Margaret turned to us and said authoritatively,

"Now that's how you play rhythm!"

Unsurprisingly, we found out later that Margaret was a professional pianist and a long-time music teacher. We have since added triplets to our repertoire of rhythm patterns for drum circles. We also learned from this music teacher that one of the most enjoyable parts of drumming together is also singing together. Once we have spent 20 or 30 minutes playing various rhythms, we often invite the group to sing an old favorite and we play the drums to accompany our singing. Before long, participants are calling out songs to sing and we all join in as we sing and drum together.

Managing costs

One of the concerns that administrations of long-term care homes and adult day centers have is the cost of providing instruments for a drum circle. For establishments that cannot afford to buy frame drums or African drums, there are some inexpensive and relatively simple alternatives. Part of Tom Gill's drumming program includes information about how to recreate drums from everyday found objects. One of his examples involves turning large plastic paint containers upside down and, on the bottom rim, inserting four tennis balls. The tennis balls will keep the drum off of the ground so that sound can escape the plastic container and the balls also keep the drum steady.

Gill has also created frame drums using packing tape stretched across a hollow box.

An ancient DNA

No matter what kinds of drums are used, drum circles can be created in intentional communities and in families. They are wonderful opportunities to have various age groups come together in an engaging activity. Children, grandchildren, and friends can join the person with dementia in making rhythm. There doesn't have to be any level of expertise; there only has to be the willingness to try something new and the desire to have fun. There is absolutely something magical that happens when people drum together. It is an ancient activity that is deep in our DNA. When we share a beat together we are signaling that we see each other and hear each other, and in so doing we are truly connecting.

At the end of every drum circle, we encourage the participants to play a rumble. This is when people beat the drum anyway they like: fast, slow, loudly, softly. The rumble usually only lasts for about a minute and then the facilitator gives the group the signal to stop. We then go around the circle and thank the drummers for joining us. It is often the case that people who came to the circle reluctantly or were showing little interest to join the group are now smiling and talking and very alive in the moment.

And this is what it is all about: our goal is that participants leave the drum circle feeling energized, smiling, having bonded with others in the circle, and maybe walking with a little more confidence, with a little spring in their step.

> If a man does not keep pace with his companions, perhaps, it is because he hears a different drummer. Let him step to the music which he hears, however measured or far away. (Henry David Thoreau)

Chapter Seven

Just Sing Your Song

JACKIE'S STORY

When we arrived at the long-term care home that morning, Jackie was screaming and screaming. The staff were all trying their very best to calm her, talking soothingly to her, trying to redirect her, interest her in something, and help her calm down. We had been working with Jackie for several months in a program we were creating at the home in which she lived. We visited the home once a week, working directly with people living with dementia while staff assisted us and observed us. We also held teaching seminars for the staff throughout the time we worked at this home. We saw the staff employing many of the techniques that we had taught them to help calm Jackie, but nothing was working.

We remembered that the week before, Jackie was one of the best singers in a group sing-along that we held. She was particularly good at recalling some of the old hymns we were singing. As the situation grew more desperate, we began to sing one of the hymns we sang with Jackie the week before.

Jackie stopped screaming and watched us closely. As we finished the first couple of lines, Jackie joined in the singing. When we began the second verse, she began to sing with us in a strong alto harmony. Jackie sank down on the couch, folded her hands, and smiled at us as the song came to a close. She asked us to sing another song with her. All of her fear and anxiety were gone. Jackie was perfectly calm and happy. It was as if a switch had been turned off the moment she heard the first few bars of that hymn.

Later we met Jackie's son and he told us that his mother had been a choir director at their church for most of her adult life. With this knowledge, we brought in a hymnal with us when we visited Jackie (remember to put something meaningful into a person's hands). We created a game with her. We would begin to sing the beginning notes or words of a hymn and Jackie would tell us the name of the song after just a few notes or words. She would often go on to sing the entire hymn.

When we brought the hymnal into the long-term care home to work with Jackie, we noticed that a group of people would gather around us and listen to Jackie guess the hymns and sing the songs. The Montessori Method teaches us to follow the person, to go where their interest lies, to talk about what they want to discuss, to let the person or people we work with lead the way. We made copies of the hymns in large print and placed the songs in binders. We would hand out the binders to several people in the home and play *Name that Hymn* with a group of people. Without fail, the group would begin to sing the hymns after someone guessed the name.

Montessori also teaches us to create extensions for exercises. These are simply the natural outgrowth of an activity. In this case, the extension for *Name that Hymn* was the creation of a choir in the long-term care home. This was not a formal choir; rather, we would ask anyone who wandered by while we were singing and accept anyone who wanted to join in. As we did in the elder reading circle and drum circles, we placed the chairs in a circle with someone counting off the beat for each hymn. One day, as we were singing with the choir, Jackie suddenly stood up and went to the center of the circle. She raised her hand, giving the choir the signal to begin singing and directed us for the remainder of the song. Before we began the next hymn, Jackie stopped, a frown on her face. Jackie told us that the choir was all wrong. She directed the sopranos to sit together, then put the altos together, and instructed the bass and baritone singers to sit together. We all shuffled around while Jackie watched us. She gave us a big smile, raised her arms, and the choir, now properly seated, began to sing again.

Leading a choir is an example of how the procedural memory works and why we find it so helpful in our work connecting to people living with dementia. When Jackie heard the choir singing, she remembered how to lead them because being a choir director engages so many muscles in the body. Once Jackie began leading the choir, she remembered that the singers should be divided by their type of voice. She also began directing with a lot of emotion, and even started giving advice and suggestions to the singers. The staff reported to us that on choir days, Jackie would have a much better afternoon and evening. The joy that the music and choir directing gave Jackie lasted well beyond the activity itself.

Singing is a prime example of an activity guided by the procedural memory system. There are so many parts of the body and muscles involved in the act of singing. It is a very physical exercise and that is why it is a procedural memory activity and is, oftentimes, spared from the effects of dementia. Singing is also a very spiritual experience. It doesn't matter what the group is singing, whether hymns or pop music; singing touches our souls in a way that very few other things in life do.

Have you ever had the experience of hearing a song from your past and suddenly you're transported back to the time when you loved that music? A song can bring back very vivid and detailed memories; we can often remember where we were, what we were wearing, who was with us, and what we were feeling when we hear a much loved song. The ability for music to move us deeply is not lost when people have dementia. Songs are often the strongest of the bridges that connect us to people who may seem lost to us. Playing songs or singing songs so often bring the past and all of its complexities and heartache and beauty back to us in a deeply moving and visceral way. We have observed that people who have lost the ability to speak coherently or to speak at all can still sing. This phenomenon is useful to both family and professional carers as it is an accessible and effective tool for reaching people who may have lost the ability to communicate.

Today there are many organizations that realize the importance of singing for people living with dementia. Choirs are more commonly found now in long-term care homes, adult day centers, and memory enhancement centers. Intergenerational choirs are being established to promote understanding across generations. One of the most successful of these intergenerational choir projects was created by the Alzheimer Society London and Middlesex (ASLM), Canada. The Intergenerational Choir began in 2012 and has since spread to other groups throughout Canada. There is a growing body of research that speaks to the efficacy of different age groups singing together. When people living with dementia are joined by younger people, there is a special bond that grows between these two groups. The younger people help their elders follow the music and the elders help the younger people understand the role that music can play in creating bonds between people, even people that seemingly have very little in common.

The ASLM created a documentary film of their first Intergenerational Choir. If you go to their website[1] you can watch the film there. It is a remarkable film showing the choir singing together as well as interviews with the teenagers who were part of the project and the elders with dementia who joined them in forming the choir. One of the most moving parts of the documentary is when a very well-known choral conductor, Ken Fleet, conducts the choir in its last song, "You'll Never Walk Alone." Mr. Fleet throws his whole body into directing the choir. It is quite obvious that he is a highly skilled and passionate choir director. Ken Fleet is interviewed after directing the choir and tells the interviewer that he also has dementia. He struggles with finding the right words but Mr. Fleet says something so profound and so beautiful at the end of the interview:

"I get up every day and try to get everyone to sing their song. Whatever it is, just sing your song!"

Kathy McNaughton, the music director of the local Medway High School and present leader of the Intergenerational Choir Project, reports that:

> At the Alzheimer Society of London and Middlesex, we offer several different Social Recreation Programs. In the past, one program triggered ideas about an Intergenerational Choir. This past program offered our clients the opportunity to create a scrapbook with one of our volunteers to assist our clients in telling their story. Over time, observing the impact of how much the clients enjoyed the music aspect of the program, it also became evident it had enhanced storytelling and reminiscing.

---

1   https://alzheimerlondon.ca

The idea continued to develop by involving not only our clients, but students and older adults as well. Medway High School music program brought on board Jeff Beynon as music director. The project was researched by Western University's faculty of education. During this research, the benefits of intergenerational music on clients with dementia showed to be tremendously positive. Now, in 2018 we are beginning our 30th session of the Intergenerational Choir, with an average of 90 members per session and now under the direction of Kathy McNaughton, Medway High Schools Music Director.[15]

Kathy brings a special presence when the Intergenerational Choir gathers on Thursdays in the Chapel at the Sisters of St. Joseph. Her warm smile and engaging laughter make all of our participants feel welcome. When Kathy chooses the music for each session, she tries to include a combination of a few things. As Kathy states:

First of all, I will pick a few familiar songs from each of the generations involved. When we started this seven years ago, we were picking WWII songs for our more mature choir members, but I have noticed that our clients from the Alzheimer's Society are getting younger and relate better to songs from The Beatles, The Beach Boys, Elvis Presley, etc. For the high school students, I will pick songs that they have performed at school before. We discovered during our first year of the project that, after only one session, the Alzheimer Society clients remembered songs that were otherwise new to them. The next session we could then use that song as a familiar selection. This was very exciting to discover. People with dementia can learn new music and will also remember that music over a period of time. And finally, over the last thirteen sessions, we have found two pieces that have become part of our tradition. "You'll Never Walk Alone" and "Blessings." Regarding the order the pieces are rehearsed and performed, we always start with a piece that is familiar, fairly upbeat and well loved by all. This session, that song is "Sentimental Journey." When compiling the music, the singers' booklets are placed in rehearsal order so that singers can simply turn the page for the next piece. At first, members will sing mainly the melody, and as rehearsals progress, harmonies are added, nuances are encouraged, dynamics are rehearsed and watching the conductor is expected, just as in any choir.[16]

The high school students bring another layer to our Intergenerational Choir. Kathy tells us each year that the students gain so much from this experience. They have the opportunity to demonstrate their leadership ability and develop friendships with people who have become a "grandparent" figure. The choir members enjoy jokes, family stories, chatting about the students' day, and their future plans. Kathy mentioned that the students also learn about people dealing with dementia, the difficulties they face, and also get to know their families and caregivers. Several students discover possibilities for their future careers after being involved in the choir. Kathy explains that, "I believe that the most important thing that the students get out of the program is a sense of empathy. The students are more sensitive, insightful and kind having been involved in the choir."

As the music director of the Intergenerational Choir, Kathy has a number of impactful stories relating to her experiences, which she shared with the ASLM, as follows:

One student that started the program with us made the decision that she would apply to study health sciences with the hope of becoming a doctor. Her long-term goal is to research the brain and diseases of the brain. The husband in one couple had been diagnosed with Alzheimer's disease and had also suffered from a stroke. The combination of these two things left him quiet, fearful and far less communicative with his family and wife. After his third choir rehearsal he asked his wife to dance with him in the kitchen, something they used to do before his diagnosis and the strokes.

There are so many stories from our Thursday evening rehearsals. After rehearsal, older partners will often get together with students for dinner or coffee. Many of our caregivers talk about their family member being in a happier mood after a rehearsal.

I enjoyed the Intergenerational Choir for many of the same reasons other students, caregivers, and people with Alzheimer's disease also enjoyed it. Not only was I able to witness both the short-term and long-term effects that music has on a person with Alzheimer's disease, but this choir also allowed me to gain a new perspective on the human experience. I loved interacting and creating intergenerational relationships through the conversations I had before, during, and after rehearsals. It is incredible to watch people's faces light up when they are given the opportunity to teach a younger generation about their passions and fondest memories. I enjoyed hearing experiences, anecdotes, and advice from the older generation as it fostered a connection that allowed me to view the human experience with a refreshing perspective. I enjoyed watching the immediate and long-term impact the choir had on people's emotions. The moment we began singing, there was an immediate, noticeable surge in spirit, happiness and memory. Some of my fondest memories were the comments and comedic anecdotes that we shared in between songs, most of which were forgotten memories and emotions that were not present at the start of rehearsal.

When we asked Alicia, a graduate of Medway High School, what her favorite song was, her response was very heartfelt and profound. Alicia remarked,

> Everyone has a different emotion and memory associated with my favorite song. For some, "You'll Never Walk Alone" reminded them of loss. For others, it was bittersweet, reminding them of their high school graduation in 1960. Singing this song, I have never felt so loved and connected to a group of people, despite not truly knowing any of them too well. No matter what memory one may associate with this song, or whether one has an associated memory at all, everyone is united in singing the words "you'll never walk alone." All of our unique experiences, individual emotions and identities were united by lyrics proclaiming a message everyone longs to hear. For those experiencing a hardship of any kind, whether it be Alzheimer's disease or not, the idea that someone will always be caring for you or "walking beside you" is incredibly moving. The idea that no one is ever truly alone is an important, and beautiful sentiment to remember.

Some of the people involved in researching the Intergenerational Choir report the following:

> There is a growing body of evidence that musical interventions have the temporary capacity to evoke emotions, influence mood, reduce emotional and behavioral disturbances, relieve pain, and improve quality of life in persons with dementia. While there is literature that describes the

role of music listening, sing-alongs, and other activities as therapies for persons with Alzheimer's disease [AD], there is little in the literature about the role of new learning through singing for those with AD. In this session, we report on a study of an innovative and collaborative intergenerational choral program that brings together persons with AD, their caregivers, high school students and their music teachers. We articulate the role that the choir plays in providing new learning opportunities for persons with AD; music and health education for adolescent students; respite, reunion, and learning opportunities for caregivers; and, professional and personal development for music educators... A result of the success of this choral program in the aforementioned areas, is that it has been shared and developed in centers across Ontario, and even to Norway.

Along with the efficacy of social bonding and new learning evidenced in group singing, research has shown that organic changes to the body may occur when groups of people sing together. Dr. Anna Haensch, Assistant Professor in the Department of Mathematics and Computer Science at Duquesne University, Pittsburgh, Pennsylvania, wrote an article about the change in heartbeats when people sing together:

> Lifting voices together in praise can be a transcendent experience, unifying a congregation in a way that is somehow both fervent and soothing. But is there actually a physical basis for those feelings? To find this out, researchers of the Sahlgrenska Academy at the University of Gothenburg in Sweden studied the heart rates of high school choir members as they joined their voices. The findings, published in *Frontiers in Neuroscience*, confirm

that choir music has calming effects of the heart—especially when sung in unison. Using pulse monitors attached to the singers' ears, the researchers measured the changes in the choir members' heart rates as they navigated the intricate harmonies of a Swedish hymn. When the choir began to sing, their heart rates slowed down.[17]

"When you sing the phrases, it is a form of guided breathing," says project leader and musicologist, Bjorn Vickhoff, of Sahlgrenska Academy. "You exhale on the phrases and breathe in between the phrases," Vickhoff explains, "[and] when you exhale, the heart slows down."

Vickhoff further states that it took almost no time at all for the singers' heart rates to become synchronized. The read-out from the pulse monitors starts as a jumble of jagged lines, but quickly becomes a series of uniform peaks. The heart rates fall into a shared rhythm guided by the song's tempo.

"The members of the choir are synchronizing externally with the melody and the rhythm, and now we see it has an internal counterpart. It's a beautiful way to feel. You are not alone but with others who feel the same way," Vickhoff says.

So while singing is a fun, social bonding experience, according to recent research, it can also calm and synchronize the heartbeats of the singers and can open up new possibilities for learning. Because of the multitude of benefits, we strongly encourage the staff and family members at every long-term care home, adult day center, and memory enhancement unit where we work to introduce group singing for elders with dementia. Sing-alongs, choirs of all descriptions, musical games (*Name that Tune, Name that Hymn*) are very powerful tools to connect people who have dementia with others. Singing in a group also provides people with the opportunity to express their emotions in a way that many cannot with words. It doesn't matter if people cannot carry a tune or if they are behind the beat or sing the wrong words, just sing anyway and take notice of the benefits for all involved.

If I cannot fly, then let me sing! (Stephen Sondheim)

Chapter Eight

Poetry Circles

Older generations were taught to read and memorize poetry when they were in school, as poetry was an important part of the curriculum. Because our elders were taught poetry, we have found that this is an art form that is quite familiar to them and one that they enjoy. Our poetry program for people living with dementia has two equal and important branches to it: one is reading poetry aloud together; the second is writing poems together. Once again, our poetry program can be used in both intentional communities and family homes.

Reading poems

To begin our poetry circle, we place several chairs in a circle. The circle can be as small as three or four participants and as large as 20 people. Or you can simply sit and read poetry aloud with one other person. We have run small and large poetry reading circles and find that both work.

We create books of poetry in large print (18+ point) and place the poems in binders. We often decorate these books with photos to help illustrate the poems. If the poem is short, then one person reads the entire poem. If the poem is more than one page long, we have one participant read one page of the poem and then move on to the next reader, and so on. After the poem is read aloud, we start a conversation about the poem. We use open-ended questions to prompt discussion. Here is an example of a poem we've used successfully:

The Lamplighter by Robert Louis Stevenson

My tea is nearly ready and the sun has left the sky;
It's time to take the window to see Leerie going by;
For every night at teatime and before you take your seat,
With lantern and with ladder he comes posting up the street.

Now Tom would be a driver and Maria go to sea,
And my papa's a banker and as rich as he can be;
But I, when I am stronger and can choose what I'm to do,
Oh Leerie, I'll go round at night and light the lamps with you!

For we are very lucky, with a lamp before the door,
And Leerie stops to light it as he lights so many more;
And O! before you hurry by with ladder and with light,
O Leerie, see a little child and nod to him tonight!

As previously mentioned, this poem is reproduced in 18+ point and there would be a picture of a lamplighter in the beginning of the poem. Because the poem is short, only one person would read it.

Some of the open-ended questions we might ask the group include:

- What was the job of the lamplighter?

- Why do you think the child in the poem wants to be a lamplighter?

- Does anyone here remember when the street lights had to be lit by a lamplighter?

- When you were a child was there a particular job you wanted to do when you grew up?

We often use classic poetry and poets. We look for poems that tend to be shorter and have obvious themes and meaning. Robert Louis Stevenson is a Scottish poet who wrote in the late 1800s, but his poetry strikes a chord with older people, some of whom remember reading his poems in school.

Another poet we often use is an American writer, John Ciardi. His poems tend to be short and funny and clever. He was born in 1916 and died in 1986, hitting the peak of popularity in the 1950s and 1960s. Here is an example of one of his poems:

About the Teeth of Sharks by John Ciardi

The thing about a shark is—teeth.
One row above, one row beneath.

Now take a close look. Do you find
It has another row behind?

Still closer-here, I'll hold your hat.
Has it a third row behind that?

Now look in and...look out! Oh my.
I'll never know now! Well, goodbye.

This poem has rhyming couplets that make it fun to read aloud. It is clever, funny, entertaining, and easy to understand. After someone reads this poem aloud, we have a discussion about the poem. We never know what twists and turns the conversations will take, and that's just fine. As facilitators, we let the discussion go where it will and follow the participants.

Another source we use for our poetry reading circles are old and very familiar nursery rhymes. Some of these rhymes seem quite sinister when examined closely, so we try to stay away from those. "Rock-a-Bye-Baby" and "Humpty-Dumpty" are two examples of rhymes that are rather dark in nature. Instead, we use nursery rhymes that are fun and easily understood. Here is an example of a nursery rhyme we often use:

As I Was Going to St. Ives

As I was going to St. Ives
I met a man with seven wives,
Each wife had seven sacks,
Each sack had seven cats,
Each cat had seven kits:
Kits, cats, sacks and wives,
How many were there going to St. Ives?

We will then ask questions such as:

- Does anyone know where St. Ives is?

- What pictures do you see in your mind when you hear this poem?

- What do you suppose the writer of this nursery rhyme was trying to teach children?

As with all of the arts that we use in our Montessori Method, the purpose of the poetry reading circle is to find a way for people living with dementia to connect with their peers, caregivers, and families. We know that these connections may not last for long, but for just that moment that we are laughing or talking about a poem, that is a connection and a moment of real joy.

We mentioned the use of classic poems, humorous poems, and nursery rhymes, but we also look for more serious poems that might speak to the participants in our poetry reading circles. We will often use poems that resonate with older people, or poems that may address their present struggles and their past glories. An example of this kind of poetry is taken from the last stanza of Alfred, Lord Tennyson's famous poem, "Ulysses:"

Old age hath yet his honour and his toil;
Death closes all: but something ere the end,
Some work of noble note, may yet be done,
Not unbecoming men that strove with Gods.
The lights begin to twinkle from the rocks:
The long day wanes: the slow moon climbs: the deep
Moans round with many voices. Come, my friends,
'Tis not too late to seek a newer world.
Push off, and sitting well in order smite
The sounding furrows; for my purpose holds
To sail beyond the sunset, and the baths
Of all the western stars, until I die.
It may be that the gulfs will wash us down:
It may be we shall touch the Happy Isles,
And see the great Achilles, whom we knew.
Tho' much is taken, much abides; and tho'
We are not now that strength which in old days

Moved earth and heaven, that which we are, we are;
One equal temper of heroic hearts,
Made weak by time and fate, but strong in will
To strive, to seek, to find, and not to yield.

This poem, in particular, can lead to some remarkable conversations. Before we begin reading, we explain to the group who Achilles is and what the term "Happy Isles" mean. After the reading, whatever meaning the group finds in this poem is completely up to the participants. We have found that many older people deeply understand the lines, "Tho' much is taken, much abides; and tho' we are not now that strength which in old days moved earth and heaven, that which we are, we are." There is often a great comfort for the group in these particular lines.

There are, of course, many classic poems from which to choose. Many well-known and beloved poems of famous writers are very light in their approach. A good example of this is Hilaire Belloc's poem, "The Early Morning."

The moon on the one hand, the dawn on the other;
The moon is my sister; the dawn is my brother.
The moon on my left and the dawn on the right.
My brother, good morning; my sister, good night.

This is a lovely poem that many people can relate to, the coming of dawn and the ending of night. It can also be read as a metaphor for the passage of time, the ending of a life, and the beginning of a new life, death, and birth. An interesting and simple conversation starter for this poem could be, "How do you feel when you watch the sun coming up?" Or, conversely, "How do you feel when you watch the sun setting in the evening?"

Another poet that we often use in our poetry reading circles is William Wordsworth, an English poet who was born in 1770 and died in 1850. He wrote many poems about nature. We find that his poetry is very popular with older people. In the following poem, Wordsworth writes about daffodils. This is a wonderful poem to read aloud in early spring with a vase full of daffodils on the table:

I Wandered Lonely as a Cloud

I wandered lonely as a cloud
That floats on high o'er vales and hills,
When all at once I saw a crowd,
A host, of golden daffodils;
Beside the lake, beneath the trees,
Fluttering and dancing in the breeze.

Continuous as the stars that shine
And twinkle on the Milky Way,
They stretched in never-ending line
Along the margin of a bay:
Ten thousand saw I at a glance,
Tossing their heads in sprightly dance.

The waves beside them danced; but they
Out-did the sparkling waves in glee:
A poet could not but be gay,
In such a jocund company:
I gazed—and gazed—but little thought
What wealth the show to me had brought:

For oft, when on my couch I lie
In vacant or in pensive mood,
They flash upon that inward eye

Which is the bliss of solitude;
And then my heart with pleasure fills,
And dances with the daffodils.

It should be noted that the work of peers, people of the same generation, and amateur poets can also speak directly to the heart of older people. Because so many older people were exposed to poetry at a young age, a surprising number of people in this generation write poetry themselves. We were very fortunate to be given a book of poems by a woman, Evelyn Pittenger, who lived a rather quiet life in a small town in Indiana. The book was not formally published. The poems were collected by her family. Within these simple poems there lies an entire life—a life of love and loss, everyday chores, special moments and, as she aged, poems filled with poignant remembering. Here is one of those poems:

First Kiss by Evelyn Grisso Pittenger

She was a lass of fifteen
He was but one year older
She was, oh, so very shy
He was a bit bolder.
He walked her home that evening,
The stars were shining bright.
And when they reached her doorstep
He gently kissed her goodnight.
Her heart was thumping madly
As he turned and walked away.
That was over sixty years ago
But she remembers to this day.

I was once that shy young girl.
And now I like to reminisce
About the days when I was young
And remember my first kiss.

This is a very simple poem but it expresses so much emotion and tenderness. It is a sure-fire conversation starter. Usually, the only open-ended question the facilitator needs to ask is: "Who has a memory of their first kiss?" And we're away. There are so many memories and feelings that come pouring out of the group, both men and women, remembering their first kiss.

Evelyn wrote many poems, but the following work is the perfect companion piece to her "First Kiss" poem:

Solitary Meal by Evelyn Grisso Pittenger

I set the table for two
As I had done for years.
Coffee in your grandpa cup
A bouquet to add some cheer.
I watched the coffee grow cold
In your grandpa cup.
Tears rolled down my cheeks.
I tried to wipe them up.
Why did I set the table
The way I used to do?
I think the only reason was
I'm lonesome for you.

While this is a more somber poem, it is also a vivid portrait of honest emotion. Sometimes when we're interacting with people living with dementia, there is a tendency to sugar-coat things, to try and make life and all of its crazy quilt of emotions a little simpler for older people. While it is a good thing to help people with dementia minimize their anxiety and frustration, we don't need to hide away real, raw emotion. These are people who have lived a long life and faced hardship and loss as we all do. Rather than pretend that these difficulties never happened in their lives, it is important to find ways to help them cope with feelings of isolation, loss, and sadness. It has been our experience that poetry is enormously helpful in dealing with all kinds of emotions. This is, after all, what poetry is designed to do, to help us try and understand the patterns in our lives.

The final category of poetry that we use in our poetry reading circles are those poems written by that famous poet, Anonymous. For some unknown reason, there seem to be a lot of poems out in the world that no one has ever claimed. Here is one example of an excellent poem that has not been claimed by its author:

> The sun it shines, regardless,
> The grass it grows, oblivious,
> The water it sits, fathomless.
> The moon it reflects, lovingly,
> The tree it stands, determinedly,
> The sand it moves, impulsively.
> Time is a constant, unstoppable,
> Space is vast, incalculable,
> Life is a gift, remarkable.

This poem can lead to a lot of discussion beginning with the question: "Why does the poet say that life is a gift, that life is remarkable?"

Here is another anonymous poem. This one is both thought-provoking and amusing:

Let's face it.
English is a strange language.
There is no egg in the eggplant,
No ham in the hamburger,
And neither pine nor apple in the pineapple.
English muffins were not invented in England.
French fries were not invented in France.

We sometimes take English for granted,
But if we examine its paradoxes we find that
Quicksand takes you down slowly,
Boxing rings are square,
And a guinea pig is neither from Guinea nor is it a pig.

If writers write, how come fingers don't fing.
If the plural of tooth is teeth,
Shouldn't the plural of phone booth be phone beeth?
If the teacher taught,
Why didn't the preacher praught.

If a vegetarian eats vegetables,
What the heck does a humanitarian eat!?
Why do people recite at a play,
Yet play at a recital?
Park on driveways and
Drive on parkways?

You have to marvel at the unique lunacy

Of a language where a house can burn up as
It burns down,
And in which you fill in a form
By filling it out,
And a bell is only heard once it goes!

English was invented by people, not computers,
And it reflects the creativity of the human race
(Which of course isn't a race at all.)

That is why
When the stars are out they are visible,
But when the lights are out they are invisible.
And why it is that when I wind up my watch
It starts.
But when I wind up this poem
It ends.

There is a rich field of poetry from which to choose and there are many types of poetry from which we can draw: classic poems, children's nursery rhymes, humorous poems, poems written by amateurs, and anonymous poems. It has been our experience that reading poetry together brings people closer to each other and closer to their own memories and emotions.

Writing poems

The second branch of our poetry circle activity is writing poems together in a group. To create these poems, everyone sits in a circle. The facilitator brings different objects for the group to hold (this is the Montessori principle of putting something meaningful in people's hands in order to prime the pump of memory). The objects can be things that relate to the present season or an upcoming holiday. Or, the objects can be taken from nature. Once the group has handled the objects, the facilitator takes up pen and paper and offers the group a starting line of poetry. This beginning line can be related to the objects brought to the group or it could be about the weather, or anything.

Once the facilitator begins the poem, the participants sitting in the poetry circle are invited to contribute a line, which the leader then writes down. If a person doesn't want to participate or isn't able to think of a line to contribute, they can say "pass" and the leader will choose the next person in the group. We don't want to intimidate or frustrate any participant, so we don't push people to contribute.

Here is an example of a poem that a large group of people living in a dementia unit wrote together. It was a beautiful spring day and the members of the poetry circle were sitting outside on the porch of a memory enhancement center. We had brought in some beautiful spring flowers for the group to pass around. After the flowers were examined by everyone we started the poem with this line: *It is a beautiful day today.* Then we went around the circle, asking people if they would like to contribute to the poem. The group wrote the following poem:

The Ladies on the Porch

It is a beautiful day today
The sun is a yellow gold
I would get up and dance but I'm too old.

Oh, let's face it. We're all old.
You're not old, I'm older than you.
Yes, you are but we can still enjoy this sky of blue.

Let's be grateful we can sit on this porch.
Yes! With all these flowers growing from the ground.
And glory shone all around!

The women who were sitting on the porch that morning, who wrote this poem together, were in different places in their respective dementia journeys. There were some women who didn't want to contribute but who nevertheless stayed in the circle to hear the poem being developed. The first stanza has a rhyme at the end of the second and third lines. This seemed to happen quite by accident. Interestingly, once the rhyming pattern was established, the group kept the same pattern going (rhyming the last words in the second and third lines). This doesn't always happen. Many of the poems we create don't have any rhymes in them at all. We are only the facilitators, writing down whatever someone in the circles says.

"The Ladies on the Porch" poem had another very interesting aspect to it. One woman, Cynthia, kept passing on her turn as we went around the circle asking people to contribute a line. We could see that Cynthia was taking this exercise very seriously but she kept saying "pass" when it came to her turn. We were trying to figure out how to end the poem when Cynthia suddenly became very animated.

"I've got it! I've got it!" Cynthia closed her eyes and clasped her hands together and recited the line, "And glory shone all around!"

The participants in the circle clapped when Cynthia finally contributed her line. It was the perfect ending to our poem.

John Killick is a Scottish poet who has been working in the field of dementia for over 20 years. He was a teacher for many years, working in adult education. Mr. Killick worked as an educator in prisons and as a writer in residence in a women's prison and hospice before he began his career working with older people. He now concentrates on writing with people who have dementia, and notes that, "Poetry is an engaging and inclusive activity for older people that can help develop memory, imagination and identity." Killick has written several books about the use of poetry in dementia care. His most recent book, *Poetry and Dementia: A Practical Guide,*[18] is filled with examples of the poetry he has used for years when he works with people living with dementia. He, too, helps people with dementia create group poems. He also helps people write one-on-one poetry. Some of these poems are simply astonishing. Killick states that the best way to elicit poetry from people living with dementia is to learn how to be a good listener and to not be afraid of silences. He explains that, "Many people are not comfortable with silence, and feel the need to fill it with chatter, however inconsequential. This has to be resisted. Somehow you have to learn to hold back and wait."[19] Here is an example of a beautiful one-on-one poem spoken by a Welsh farmer who had not spoken aloud in a very long time. As he sat and gazed at a field of sheep, he spoke these words:

A Good Life

We were farmers, sheep and cattle,
At our farm, Ty'r Capel
Pen Groesffordd, east of Brecon.

I had a brother, Glanville,
And a sister, Mary.
One or two others as well.

The family grew.
Whenever we married,
We had no end of children.
Three hundred acres
In a sheltered valley,
Lots of fields.

We spoke Welsh from our mother's knee,
Went to chapel quite regular,
Took the sheep to market.

It was a good life,
Though some might say small.
I wouldn't have had any other.

This poem came to be because the person listening to the farmer waited patiently and quietly. It is true that time is often in short supply for carers. But if we can slow down, if only for a few minutes, and wait for them to speak and then listen deeply to what is being said, we may be given a gift like this poem from a usually silent Welsh sheep farmer.

As we've stated before, we're often surprised in this dementia work. One of our most remembered and treasured surprises came one day when we were holding one of our poetry reading circles. A son of one of the participants came to visit his mother. He was a construction worker and came to visit her that day wearing his overalls and boots. He stopped dead and stood very still listening to us reading aloud a poem from the Irish poet, W.B. Yeats. The poem was this classic:

The Song of Wandering Aengus

I went out to the hazel wood
Because a fire was in my head
And I cut and peeled a hazel wand
And hooked a berry with a thread
And when white moths were on the wing
And moth-like stars were flickering out
I dropped a berry in a stream
And caught a little silver trout.
When I had laid it on the floor

I went to blow the fire aflame
But something rustled on the door
And someone called me by my name.
It had become a glimmering girl
With apple blossoms in her hair
Who called me by my name and ran
And faded through the brightening air.

Though I am old with wandering
Through hollow lands and hilly lands
I will find out where she has gone
And kiss her lips and take her hands
And walk among long dappled grass
And pluck till time and times are done
The silver apples of the moon,
The golden apples of the sun.

As we neared the end of the poem, the construction worker stood, eyes closed and began reciting with us, from memory, the lines, "And pluck till time and times are done, the silver apples of the moon, the golden apples of the sun."

We would have never guessed that this tough looking man would know and love this poem. We learned that day to always include everyone in our poetry reading circles. You never know who will be touched by a poem.

Poetry is when an emotion has found its thought and the thought has found words. (Robert Frost)

Chapter Nine

Video Diaries

JO-JO'S STORY

Jo-Jo was a woman in her fifties who had lived at home with her mother all of her life. When her mother was diagnosed with Alzheimer's, Jo-Jo went with her mom to the long-term care home where they could both be cared for. Jo-Jo had never spoken and had been diagnosed as mentally retarded when she was a child. She had never gone to school nor had she had any sort of work life or social life. Jo-Jo's way of getting attention was to head butt people. She helped her mom around the house and the farm where they both lived until they were admitted to the care home.

When we began to interact with Jo-Jo in the Alzheimer's unit of the long-term care home, we soon realized that she was deaf. She had never been diagnosed as having hearing loss. Jo-Jo was delighted with the simple sign language that we taught her and was soon able to tell the staff when she was hungry, thirsty, in pain, or upset. Jo-Jo loved technology and was fascinated by the camera we were using to film video diaries. (This was before camera phones and we were still using a hand-held video camera to make films.)

One day, we handed the camera to Jo-Jo and showed her the button to push to start filming. She started to moan and cry when we gave her the camera. One of the carers in the home rushed over to see what was upsetting Jo-Jo. But it soon became apparent to all of us that Jo-Jo was crying because she was so happy. She learned how to move the lens in for close-ups and how to pan the room to give the video context. The only problem with Jo-Jo's films was that she moaned with happiness the entire time she filmed.

Another piece of equipment that fascinated Jo-Jo was a pen we used in our work. When we saw that Jo-Jo was very interested in the pen, we gave it to her. When one of the nurses at the care home accidentally picked up Jo-Jo's pen and took it to the nurses' station, Jo-Jo stood by anxiously on one foot and then another, pointing to the pen, and becoming very agitated. Finally, the nurse realized her mistake and returned the pen to Jo-Jo. We taught Jo-Jo how to hold the pen and how to write her name. She was so thrilled to be able to write her name and practiced writing it over and over, her hand clumsily holding the cherished pen.

The last day of Jo-Jo's life she helped us film one of our videos (moaning with joy the entire time), had lunch, and afterwards sat down at her table to practice writing. The staff found her slumped over her work. Jo-Jo died instantly of a massive heart attack. For the last few months of her life, Jo-Jo was involved in learning to communicate with sign language, learning how to make films, and learning to write. Jo-Jo spent the majority of her life locked away from other people. She was loved and cared for but she had no way to communicate, other than head butting. Holding a camera while other people told their stories was one way that Jo-Jo could communicate and play an important role in her community.

We wanted to begin this chapter on video diaries with the story of Jo-Jo, although she was never herself in a video diary, as she had no way to tell her own story. But she did help tell the stories of other people in the intentional community where she lived the last years of her life. Whenever we film someone for a video diary or when we speak about video diaries, we will always remember Jo-Jo and the contribution she made in sharing the stories of others, stories that she could never tell herself.

We begin the process of creating video diaries the same way we begin so much of our Montessori approach to connecting to people living with dementia: we give the person something meaningful to hold in their hands.

MARILYN'S STORY

For Marilyn, the prompt that released a lot of memories for her was a photography book of Murfreesboro, Tennessee, the town where she grew up. As Marilyn pored over the photographs in the book, she began to talk to us about her childhood there. As we filmed her remembering her hometown, Marilyn told us,

"Our dad would take us kids around the town. Murfreesboro wasn't a big town then. He would take us all around and say to us, 'Now, look at that,' and then he'd say, 'Now, you children, look at this.' Our dad wanted us to really see the world, to see it and understand what was going on."

Marilyn's eyes took on a faraway look and we could see that she was back in Murfreesboro with her siblings and her father, looking where he pointed, seeing what he saw and remembering it all so vividly.

These are the types of memories that we often capture when we film video diaries—small moments, a flash of a scene that suddenly comes alive for the person we are filming. The beauty of these video diaries is that they not only capture a memory, they also capture the person in the moment when they remember a scene from long ago.

Everyone has their own story to tell and each person has their own way of approaching the process of creating a video diary. Some people, once they begin talking, just keep going. Other people need some prompts and help along the way. We provide this assistance by asking open-ended questions. We make a point of avoiding questions that deal with facts such as, "How many years were you married?" Or, "Where were you living then?" These fact-based questions can lead to anxiety and frustration for the person with dementia. Fact-based information, as mentioned earlier, is stored in the declarative memory system. This is the memory system that tends to be greatly impacted by dementia and therefore information like dates, times, and places are very difficult to recall for people living with dementia.

The questions that we ask are designed to keep the conversation and memories flowing. We have found that questions that have to do with feelings rather than facts are the most helpful types. We won't ask what year something happened, but we will ask how the person felt when this particular event happened. As well as asking open-ended questions, we also make brief observations, such as, "I think you must have felt very happy when he asked you out," or, "That would have made me really angry if that happened to me." Just remember, *feelings* not *facts*. Although the stories vary widely from person to person, we have observed that everyone who participates in filming stories from their lives feels a joy and a peace when they are talking to the camera and telling their stories. And for us, the videographers, there is always surprise at the fascinating stories people share with us in their video diaries. Here is one of our very favorite (and most surprising) video diary stories:

PAUL'S STORY

Paul was a highly regarded scientist. He had taught in a major university and conducted important research on arable crops that had an impact on world-wide farming techniques. Knowing his life's work, we brought in small galvanized buckets containing different types of grain. We invited Paul to feel the grain again. He happily plunged his hands into the buckets, letting the showers of grain slide through his fingers. His eyes took on a dreamy look as the grain fell from his fingers back into the bucket. Then, to our amazement, Paul, the scientist began to tell us about his one great love, Sherry Sandeford, the girl who got away, the reason he never married.

As we were filming Paul talking about Sherry, his whole physical being began to change. His face became flushed and his breathing came rapidly, his eyes brightening with the memory of her. He never said why they did not make a match of it. He only told us of his great love for Sherry and of her loveliness.

Paul's video diary isn't sad. He lived a full and very productive life. But there was a wistfulness in his video. He was a man of science who never forgot his one true love. We thought when we brought in buckets of grain that Paul would talk about his work in agricultural science, but he remembered instead how he met and fell in love with Sherry. It was a remarkable experience for us to capture this more intimate aspect of Paul's life and a powerful reminder that everyone has profound stories to tell.

Our goal in creating video diaries is to capture these types of moments for people. For all of us, memory isn't usually linear, but rather often comes to us as flashes of a scene, a photograph of a moment in our mind, a feeling that is fleeting. These are the flashes of memory, the moments from a life that we hope to capture in video diaries. We try to prime the pump of memory by bringing in meaningful objects or playing music or involving people in an activity that they loved doing.

MARY'S STORY

Mary grew up and lived most of her life in the city. She told us often how she and her family would sit on the front steps of their home (the stoop, she called it) and watch the activity going on in their street. Mary replicated this stoop sitting by placing a chair outside of her bedroom door in the long-term care home and watching the activity in the hallway outside of her room. Sometimes, she would wave and engage people who passed in the hallway. Other times she would sit quietly, just watching.

We knew that Mary had been well known in her family and her neighborhood for the pies she baked. We asked Mary if she would like to join us in making some pies. Mary replied, shaking her head.

"Oh gosh, I don't remember how to do that! I wouldn't know where to begin."

We set up a table with pie dough, some blueberries, flour, sugar, and butter, a wooden board, and a rolling pin. Mary put on some latex gloves and looked carefully at all of the different things on the table. She began to sprinkle flour on the board, slapped down the pie dough, rubbed the rolling pin down with flour and began to roll out the pie dough in quick, certain movements. She then expertly rolled up the dough on the rolling pin and transferred it to the pie pan.

We filmed Mary as she made the blueberry pie, absolutely focused on the task at hand. She made a blueberry pie with a beautiful lattice crust, crimping the edges in perfect little indentations all around the edge of the pie. She stood back and sighed, a look of absolute satisfaction on her face. Mary said very little in her video diary but her expert handling of the different steps of pie making told volumes about her life as an expert baker.

When we complete each video diary, we show it to the person who was the subject of the video. The first time we showed a video diary to one of the people we filmed, we were dismayed by the reaction the video received. We had filmed Ginny as she told us the story of how she met her husband. She became very animated when she talked of how they first fell in love. When we showed Ginny the film, she shouted at us, "Who is that old woman and why is she talking about my husband? How does she know all that stuff about me and my husband? Who is she?"

Ginny was very angry and agitated, and we were just about to turn off the video when Ginny, watching herself, began to smile and nod. And then she pointed at the screen and told us, "I don't know who she is but that old lady sure got that right! She's good, isn't she?"

So we learned, the hard way, that before we show a participant their video, we tell them that they filmed this video with us, and that it is a film of them telling us some things about their lives. Upon learning to introduce each video diary, we have never had a negative response to the films again. Most people are absolutely fascinated watching themselves telling stories from their own lives. It is a wonderful experience to see their faces as they listen to the stories from their lives.

We often put music to parts of these diaries, or we film photographs from the lives we're chronicling. We also film the object or objects that prompted the memories and stories we film. We have found that video diaries are wonderful gifts to the families of people living with dementia. Grandchildren or great-grandchildren who may not remember, or who never met their grandparents, can meet them and know a little of their lives through these video diaries.

Using video diaries for training

Another benefit to making video diaries is that the videos can be a valuable training tool for frontline staff. Watching the stories of the people they care for, carers begin to form a more complete picture of each individual living under their care. Video diaries can play a very important role in building a person-centered dementia care program. Watching these diaries, we begin to understand, in a visceral way, that the people we care for are first and foremost people who have lived a long life. They have their own special memories and stories. They deserve to be honored and respected for the life they've lived and shared.

There have been some studies that research the efficacy of video diaries for people who have dementia. In an article written by Laurie Wang, the author states:

A recent study from the University of Alberta in Edmonton has found that digital diaries which include family photos and recorded details about the images can help patients with dementia recover memories and fight cognitive decline. According to the *Edmonton Sun*, participants worked with researchers to create video storytelling diaries; selecting pictures, music and narrating their creations. By delving into the project, volunteers with Alzheimer's were able to uncover memories long forgotten and in the process exercise their cognitive abilities.[20]

"As the people I worked with shaped their own stories, they were able to recall new memories. Even after they watched the story with their loved ones, some of the images would uncover more memories from the past," said Elly Park, principal investigator and assistant clinical lecturer in the Faculty of Rehabilitation Medicine's Department of Occupational Therapy.

"Sitting down with the participant to work on the five-minute story helped them think of positive memories," explained Park. "As we shared stories, deeply buried memories would surface. Creating a story with voice, images and music also gave them an emotional legacy piece." She added that people who have dementia are often scared of losing their ability to communicate. "Another participant told me, 'One of my fears is, I went through dementia with my mother and it gets bad at the end. And that's all the memories I seem to have, is all the bad stuff.' She really appreciated this opportunity to create something positive that her family could have to remember her."

Park and her team analyzed the participants' interviews about their experiences with this digital storytelling process. The results showed the impact was quite powerful in various ways. The participants thoroughly enjoyed the process of reminiscing and sharing stories, but were also astounded with what was possible when using technology and multimedia to present their stories. The team found engaging individually with each participant was a critical part of making this process enjoyable.

One of the pioneers of video diaries is award-winning videographer, Sitar Rose. After training in Social

Anthropology at the University of Edinburgh, Rose started making documentaries in 1980. She specializes in health education work and the arts, and frequently works with sensitive and difficult issues. As a community arts worker, she has facilitated adults and children to produce their own film projects and has developed a way of working creatively with film to help people with long-term physical and mental health problems.

As a specialist in creating video diaries of people living with dementia, Rose employed techniques designed to inspire conversation, such as placing something meaningful in a person's hands and then gently asking questions about the object. Sometimes she would play music that family members told her was special to the person with dementia. Other times she would film them participating in activities that they dearly loved. Watching these early forays into video diaries with people living with dementia taught us how powerful this medium can be in connecting once again to the people we care for. We will be forever grateful to Sitar Rose for leading the way in creating meaningful films of our elders, video diaries that can be shared with families and friends, videos that celebrate each person's life.

Regarding her experiences creating video diaries, or video portraits as she often calls this work, Rose notes that "these video portraits are about rediscovering the person hidden by dementia and is in no way an exposé on the effect dementia has had on the person." We have found this to be true whether we are involved in making video diaries or using any of the arts projects chronicled in this book. People with dementia are the people they have always been. It is up to us to find the ways and means to reach them, to "rediscover the person hidden by dementia." Rose's work in creating these video diaries gives the participants the opportunity "to express their individuality despite their difficulty in communication." Giving someone something meaningful to hold in their hands, playing much loved music, or showing them photographs from their past are proven techniques that we consider a "paradigm for connecting to people with dementia, where people can emerge productively in the process of life review."[21]

> Memories of our lives, of our works and our deeds will continue in others. (Rosa Parks)

Chapter Ten

The Lamplighters

We began this book by telling our own stories, explaining how we came to work in the dementia field. Some of you reading this book chose, as we did, to dedicate your lives to helping people living with dementia. Some of you became carers because it was thrust upon you; someone you love has been diagnosed with a form of dementia and there you are, life upended, future plans thrown out the window, sometimes feeling alone, angry, frustrated, often confused, and always tired.

While we recognize how very stressful working as a carer can be (family or professional caregiving), please know that the work you are doing, caring for the very vulnerable, makes you a hero. It doesn't make you rich, it doesn't make you better than anyone else, it doesn't make you wiser than anyone else, but this work does make you more patient, more compassionate, more loving, and more courageous. Not all of the time, not every day, but just as the person with dementia has flashes of connection, so you, too, have moments of compassion, patience, and courage. Through the exhaustion, isolation, and loss, there are those moments that are funny, that are special, that are precious. Our intention in writing this book is to help all of you find those moments of joy and triumph, however rare and

fleeting they may be. These are the moments that keep us
going, that make all of the hard work worth it.

Honesty

One of the more difficult aspects of the relationship
between people living with dementia and their carers is the
question of honesty: when the person we care for asks to
see her husband and we know that he is dead, what should
we do? If we're totally honest and tell her that her husband
is dead, that will devastate her. Should we then lie and
say that her husband is at work and will return soon? We
know that, because they have dementia, the person most
likely won't remember that we told her that her husband is
still alive. If we lie we may prevent anguish and grief, and
shouldn't that be our goal?

This is a very thorny issue, one that we've wrestled with
over the years. After much research, soul searching, and
discussion we've come down on the side of honesty, but
honesty with compassion. If a person asks us where their
spouse is and we know that they have passed away, we
answer this way: "Your husband isn't here right now. Can
you tell me some things you and your husband like to do
together?" In saying that someone's spouse or mother or
father isn't present, we are telling the truth. But then we
ask them to talk about the person they're seeking. It may
seem that we're splitting hairs but we feel very strongly that
it is important to be honest with the people we care for so
that we can preserve and respect the relationship we have
with them.

We are also straightforward when people we work
with ask us why they are doing this particular exercise
or activity. We tell them that we are all doing this work

because it helps our brains. We include ourselves in this explanation. We try very hard to work *with* people, not *for* them, just as we try very hard to speak *with* people, and not *at* them. These are goals we set for ourselves. We don't always achieve these goals (being compassionately honest, working with people and not for them), but we know that it is important to keep trying.

Positive language

Another aspect of the Montessori Method for staying connected to people living with dementia is being very mindful of the language we use. It isn't easy, but it is very important to strive to always use positive language. We have observed that this one simple change in our speech and our attitude can make the entire day much more pleasant for everyone. Instead of saying, "You can't go to the store unless you have your shower first," we try to remember to say, "After you take a shower, then we'll go to the store." The first one sounds like a command and carries a negative connotation with it. The second is more like a suggestion, a statement of fact, something to look forward to.

Along with the use of positive language, we try to match our speed of speech and movement to the speed of the person we're caring for. We understand that time is often in short supply in caregiving, but giving someone just a few more minutes to button their own shirt or cut up their own food gives the person with dementia the opportunity to demonstrate some independence. The feeling that one has some control in life creates confidence and a feeling of wellbeing.

These suggestions for more positive dementia care may seem obvious. It is the small steps that build the Montessori approach to positive dementia care. Remembering to introduce ourselves when we enter a room; making sure that we first stand in front of the person in a wheelchair and explain to them why we're moving them. We also try to be mindful that we don't toss off some conversational piece over our shoulder as we're walking away, and nor should we talk about the person with dementia in front of them, as though they are not present. These seemingly small considerations go a long way to help people living with dementia feel less anxious and more included in the everyday life of the intentional community or the family home.

Giving choices

Another aspect of building a positive relationship in dementia care is to give the people we care for some choices during the day. These can be quite simple, like, "Would you like blue cheese dressing on your salad or vinaigrette?" We know that the executive function of the declarative memory system is often damaged in people who have dementia and, because of that, it may be difficult for them to make choices. But, like everything else in life, if we give people the opportunity to practice making simple choices, this task can become easier for them. Giving someone a choice, large or small, gives them a sense of autonomy, a feeling of dignity and respect. When someone feels that they are in control, they are less likely to become anxious or frustrated.

Applying the Montessori Method to person-centered care

Part of our work in the dementia field is holding workshops and teaching seminars for carers, families, medical staff, and friends of people who have dementia. We've summed up some important points of the application of the Montessori Method in positive dementia care. Here are the major principles of the Montessori Method and its application to person-centered dementia care:

- *The environment meets the needs of the people using it.* People need to be able to move easily and safely. There should be no clutter and no busy designs on furniture, carpets, or wall coverings. Toilet seats should be of a contrasting color to the white toilet. Place settings should have contrasting colors to differentiate between plate, placemat, and table. Plants and animals should be part of the environment, as they bring a sense of home and wellbeing. Paintings should be hung so that people in wheelchairs can see them easily. PA systems should never be used in a care home or adult day centers. The people who are using the environment should be part of decisions made about the place where they live. They should be given the opportunity, whenever possible, to be included in the care of the environment, and given a sense of ownership of their intentional community.

- *Put something meaningful in a person's hands.* Use objects from nature or objects that have a deep personal attachment. This simple act helps orient people to the activity and also primes the pump of memory. It is very difficult for people living with dementia to begin a task or a discussion out of thin air; they need something concrete to help them begin.

- This is a *strength-based program*. Look for spared abilities and remaining strengths in each person. Every person has something that they can contribute. We all need a reason to get up in the morning.

- Montessori is a *comprehensive approach that is used 24/7*. It is not an activity program; it is a philosophy that encompasses the entire manner in which we build and keep relationships.

- We *follow the person with whom we are working*. Wherever the activity, exercise, or conversation goes, we follow along. We are guides, not bosses. We invite people to join us; we never insist.

- *Completing the task at hand* (beginning, middle, end) gives people a sense of accomplishment. We allow people to work on an activity or exercise as long as they wish without interrupting them.

- *No praise, no blame*. We allow people to work on an activity or exercise without judging their work. In the Montessori Method, process is much more important than product. It is the experience that matters, not the outcome.

- *Isolate the difficulty*. If a person is having problems completing an entire activity, break the work down into small steps. Some people may be able to accomplish only one step out of many, but they are still making a contribution.

- The *unique gifts of each person are recognized and celebrated*. We look for those things that people can contribute to their intentional community or their family and we celebrate their contributions.

- *Honor the beauty and strength of the human spirit*. It has been our observation that while the body may grow weaker, the spirit grows stronger. There are many gifts of wisdom, humor, and grit that older people have to share, life lessons that can benefit their friends, family, and their community.

One of the unique aspects of our Montessori Method for connecting to people with dementia is our encouragement for elders to make contributions to their intentional communities, their families, and even larger society. The German philosopher, Friedrich Nietzsche, wrote, "He who has a why to live can bear almost any how."

In other words, we all need a reason to get up in the morning.

Giving back

We've created several projects for people living with dementia that give back to different communities. The following are examples of some of the contributions that elders have made to their own community, care home or family home.

We partnered with a high school for at-risk adolescents. These young people were often abused, homeless, or had learning disabilities. The teenagers were invited to come to the care home to work on different projects with people who have dementia. Each older person was partnered with a teenager.

We created a project for them to make Thanksgiving cards to send to people in the care home, nearby hospitals, and to the elders' families. The concept was simple. We asked the elders what they were grateful for and the teenagers wrote down what the older people told them. These thoughts were written inside the card. The teenagers and elders decorated the outside of the card together by doing leaf rubbing. An autumn leaf was placed inside the card, bumpy side up. One person held the card still and their team member would rub the flat part of a Crayola (paper cover removed) over the front of the card, creating an image of the leaf.

While the two groups were working on these projects, there were many conversations going on. One young girl told an elder that she would be grateful if her family could find somewhere to live. The older person became very concerned and the two of them began talking about places where the teenager could look for help. The older person mentioned that her church often helped families and so did the local Lions Club. The time that these two groups spent together, talking about gratitude, relationships, holidays, home, was invaluable. Just being in the same space proved to be an uplifting experience for both the young people and the older people.

Another opportunity for contributing to the wider world came about when the local Alzheimer's Association asked the residents of a memory enhancement center to create artwork for a series of greeting cards. These cards would then be sold as part of a holiday fundraising project. We explained to the participants that the paintings they created would be reprinted on cards, and that these cards would be sold to raise money for the Alzheimer's Association in their town. Even though some of the people creating these paintings were themselves living with Alzheimer's, everyone enthusiastically joined in to create a painting. In that moment, the group realized that they were participating in something larger than themselves. We don't know how long this good feeling lasted, but we do know that the "halo effect" is a real phenomenon. People who are involved in meaningful work tend to have a much better time for the rest of the day.

Meaningful work

There are many types of meaningful work that can be introduced to people living with dementia. For example, one summer day we brought terracotta pots, a bag of potting soil, bee balm plants, lavender, and Sweet William flowers into a memory center. These plants are safe for people and attract bees and butterflies. Before we began to plant the flowers, we showed a short video on how monarch butterflies and certain honey bees are struggling due to environmental changes. The people in the group seemed to grasp that the flowers they were planting for the garden would help both the bees and the butterflies. That day, a husband of a woman participating in this project happened to be visiting. His wife wanted to help plant the flowers but she was having difficulty holding the small trowel. Her husband put his hand over hers and together they planted the flowers. While the group worked, they talked about the gardens they had at their home and flowers they remembered picking in their childhood. These simple projects are designed to give our elders an opportunity to contribute once again, and we have seen so many small, beautiful moments happen in the midst of these projects, like the loving hand-over-hand husband and wife team working together.

This phenomenon of being present when these meaningful moments occur has been one of the most surprising elements of our work with people living with dementia. Our mission is to be of service to people living with dementia and their families, but often we are the ones receiving gifts from the people with dementia and their carers. We honestly didn't expect that we would be the recipients of so much profound wisdom, humor, and joy. When people we meet learn about the work we do, they often say, "That seems so depressing." We smile and shake our heads and answer, "No. It isn't depressing. There's a special kind of joy working with people who are completely themselves and have a unique view of the world."

Such perceptions are centered on a larger central question:

> Can a person still be who they are if they cannot remember who they were?

After many years of working directly with people who have dementia and their carers, we have come to understand that people who have dementia are the people they always were. They are still there, the person we knew and loved. They cannot reach out to us anymore; we must be the ones who reach out to them. We have to find whatever works, whatever key there is to unlocking moments of connection, even if only for a flash of recognition, a smile, a squeeze of the hand. This is what we are meant to do, to find a way to connect.

A positive dementia experience

Looking back on our work, we realize that one of the most important contributions we have made is that we have helped define the dementia experience in much more positive terms. In the early days of our work, we heard these phrases over and over, "People with dementia are the walking dead." "Dementia is the long goodbye." "Dementia robs them of their personhood." These words are frightening and, if you let them define your life, there is nowhere to go with this kind of thinking. We are not denying that caring for someone living with dementia is a demanding, exhausting, and sometimes very lonely life. But we have seen that by changing our own attitudes to dementia, we can change how we feel about our lives, we can change how we look at the person we care for, and we can change how others view us and the people we care for. We know that this is not easy to do, but we also know that this attitude adjustment is vital in order to find some measure of happiness and peace.

Our lives are forever changed by dementia, but dementia does not have to define our lives or the lives of the people we care for. We have the power of changing the tapes that play in our heads. We have the power to make our outlook more positive, more understanding, more expansive. The person living with dementia cannot change their circumstances, nor can they change their attitudes or their outlook. As carers, we have the ability to change the course of a caregiving day by our thoughts, words, and actions. We recognize that this is a lot to ask of carers who are already exhausted and often frustrated and even angry. But, as Dr. Montessori teaches us, we isolate each difficulty, we break down what seems impossible into small steps and we try very hard to use positive language and to check our attitudes about dementia and caregiving. Even though caregiving is very challenging, it is often rewarding. We know that it may not feel like it most days, but the work you are doing is invaluable to the people you care for and invaluable to society at large. You are caring for some of the most vulnerable among us.

Thank you for your dedication, your strength, and for your loving and compassionate hearts.

In this world that can be so overwhelming, so frightening, and so dark, where we all stumble and fall, where we are often stymied by road blocks, where we sometimes lose our way, you are the lamplighters. You light our path.

Cast me not off in the time of old age: Forsake me not when my strength faileth. (Psalm 79:1)

Endnotes

1   Martin Buber (1958) *I and Thou.* New York: Charles Scribner's Sons, pp.19–22.

2   Tom Kitwood (1997) *Dementia Reconsidered: The Person Comes First.* Buckingham/Philadelphia, PA: Open University Press, p.137.

3   Maria Montessori (1949) *The Absorbent Mind.* Adyar, India: The Theosophical Publishing House, p.157.

4   Tillick, P. (1960) *Power, Love & Justice: Ontological Analysis & Ethical Applications.* Oxford: Oxford University Press, p.24.

5   Tillick, P. (1960) *Power, Love & Justice: Ontological Analysis & Ethical Applications.* Oxford: Oxford University Press, p.24.

6   William Wordsworth (1802) 'My Heart Leaps Up.'

7   L.P. Hartley (1953) *The Go-Between.* London: Hamish Hamilton.

8   G.K. Chesterton (1909) *Orthodoxy.* New York: John Lane Company, pp.153–154.

9   Ken Robinson (2009) *The Element: How Finding Your Passion Changes Everything.* New York: Penguin, p.9.

10 Tom Gill (2005) *Rhythm Adventures Exploring & Celebrating Creativity with Rhythm: A Hands-On Facilitator's Guide for Sharing Rhythm with Elders.* Milwaukee, WI: Unity Enterprises, p.2.

11 Gill (2009), ibid., p.32.

12 Gill (2009), ibid., p.34.

13 Gill (2009), ibid., p.17.

14 M. Roerdink, P.J. Bank, C.L. Peper and P.J. Beek (2011) 'Walking to the beat of different drums: Practical implications for the use of acoustic rhythms in gait rehabilitation.' *Gait Posture 33*, 4, 690–694. Available at www.ncbi.nlm.nih.gov/pubmed/21454077

15 Kathy McNaughton, Music Director. Interviewed by Jenn Pruder, Certified Therapeutic Recreation Specialist, Alzheimer Society London and Middlesex, Ontario, Canada, October 2018.

16 Carol A. Beynon, Betsy Little, Kathy McNaughton, Jeffrey G. Beynon, Jennifer M.J. Lang Hutchison and Nancy O'Regan (2016) 'Singing my way back to you: Learnings from the Intergenerational Choir Project for singers with Alzheimer's disease, their caregivers, music educators, and students.'

Alzheimer's & Dementia: The Journal of the Alzheimer's Association 12, 7, 799, July 25. Available at www.alzheimersanddementia.com/article/S1552-5260(16)31915-X/fulltext

17   Anna Haensch (2013) 'When choirs sing, many hearts beat as one.' July 10. Available at www.npr.org/sections/health-shots/2013/07/09/200390454/when-choirs-sing-many-hearts-beat-as-one

18   John Killick (2017) *Poetry and Dementia: A Practical Guide.* London and Philadelphia, PA: Jessica Kingsley Publishers, p.59.

19   Killick (2017), ibid., p.54.

20   Laurie Wang (2017) 'Digital storytelling helps people with dementia trigger memories.' *Folio* August 22, 1–2. Available at www.folio.ca/digital-storytelling-helps-people-with-dementia-trigger-memories

21   Sitar Rose (2006) 'Video portraits: Creating lasting records. *The Journal of Dementia Care 14*, 5, 23–24.

Index

activities
connecting with the past 51–2
reading 62–8
African drums 88, 95
agitation 35, 36, 48
Alzheimer Society London and
Middlesex (ASLM), Canada
100–1, 103
Alzheimer's Association 146–7
American League 51

Basho, Matsuo 54
Basting, Anne 82
Belloc, Hilaire "The Early Morning"
114
Bradford Dementia Group 25
Brenner, Karen 11
applying Montessori methods to
dementia care 13–15
building on strengths 18–19
cancer treatment 17–18
connection 19–21
reaching the unreachable 12
"We can't be brave by ourselves"
15–17
Brenner, Tom 11, 21–2
applying the Montessori
philosophy 22–4
Buber, Martin 19–20

care for the whole person 34
individual needs 34–5

carers 23–4, 139–40
applying Montessori Method to
person-centered care 33–4,
143–5
game creation 68
giving back to the community
145–7
giving choices 142
honesty 140–1
individual needs 35–6
meaningful work 147–8
positive dementia experience
149–50
positive language 141–2
taking care of the carers 52–4
Casa dei Bambini, Rome 30–1
Chesterton, G.K. *Orthodoxy 52*
choice 37–8, 142
choirs 100–8
Ciardi, John 111
"About the Teeth of Sharks"
111–12
circle meetings 86–7
communication problems 13, 16,
18
building on strengths 18–19
connecting with the past 41–2
Chet's story 50–1
exercises and activities 51–2
Helen's story 44–5
listening deeply 43–7
natural world 47–8
putting something meaningful
into someone's hands 43, 49

connecting with the past *cont.*
taking care of the carers 52–4
veterans 48–9
connection 19–21
bringing order out of chaos 35

deafness 13, 16, 127
declarative memory system 28–9,
130, 142
dementia care 11–12
applying Montessori methods
13–15
applying Montessori philosophy
22–4
care for the whole person 34
challenging behaviors 13–16
choice 37–8, 142
environment 31, 32–3, 143
honesty 140–1
positive language 36–7, 141–2
Djembe 88
drum circles 86–90
ancient DNA 96
call and response 90–1
Gary's story 85–6
hand over hand 91
Jack's story 93
managing costs 95
Margaret's story 93–5
mirroring 91
other benefits of drumming 92–5
side by side 91
triplets 94–5
verbal and non-verbal
encouragement 92

Eden Alternative® 47
empathetic identification 38–9
environment 31
serving needs of the people using
it 32–3, 143
episodic memory 29
executive function 29, 38
exercises
connecting with the past 51–2
reading 62–8

failure to initiate 37–8, 77–8
Fleet, Ken 101
fMRI (functional Magnetic
Resonance Imaging) 55
frame drums 88, 92, 95
Frost, Robert 126

gait rehabilitation 92–3
games 62–3
Category Sort 63–5
Finish the Phrase 62
joke cards 65–6
Name that Hymn 98, 107
Name that Tune 62
Trivia 66–8
Gill, Tom 87–8, 89
drumming rhythms 90–1
extra help for drum circles 91–2
home-made drums 95
Green House Project 47

Haensch, Anna 106–7
Hartley, L.P. 42
Hemingway, Ernest 84
Homer, Winslow *The Gulf Stream
80*

individual needs 34–5
carers 35–6
Intergenerational Choir, Canada
100–6

Killick, John 122–3
Kitwood, Thomas 25–6, 31, 40
common ground with Maria
Montessori 32–9

listening 43, 45–7, 54
Helen's story 44–5

McNaughton, Kathy 101–4
Montessori Method 17–18, 22
applying Montessori Method to
person-centered care 33–4,
143–5

applying Montessori philosophy 22–4
independent learners 31–2
painting 78, 83
positive language 141–2
prepared environment 30–1, 143
procedural and declarative memory systems 28–30
putting something meaningful into someone's hands 43, 49, 57, 98, 120–1, 129, 132, 136, 137, 143–4
singing 98
using materials 27–8, 29–30
Montessori, Maria 26–32, 40, 63, 149
common ground with Thomas Kitwood 32–9
MRI scans 55
muscle memory 28, 29–30

National League 51
Native American proverb 73
natural world 47–8
Nietzsche, Friedrich 145
nursery rhymes 112

painting 75–8
Billie's story 84
discussing artworks 79–80
Janie's story 75
Marilyn's story 82–3
materials 77
Maxine's story 80–1
Park, Elly 135
Parks, Rosa 137
past life 41–2
Chet's story 50–1
exercises and activities 51–2
Helen's story 44–5
listening deeply 43–7
natural world 47–8
putting something meaningful into someone's hands 43, 49
taking care of the carers 52–4
veterans 48–9

person-centered care 25–6, 39–40
applying Montessori Method to person-centered care 33–4, 143–5
Pittenger, Evelyn Grisso 116
"First Kiss" 116–17
"Solitary Meal"117–18
poetry circles 109
"A Good Life" 123–4
Anonymous "Let's face it" 119–20
Anonymous "The sun it shines, regardless" 118–19
"As I Was Going to St Ives" 112
Belloc, Hilaire "The Early Morning" 114
Ciardi, John "About the Teeth of Sharks" 111–12
Pittenger, Evelyn Grisso "First Kiss" 116–17
Pittenger, Evelyn Grisso "Solitary Meal"117–18
reading poems 109–10
Stevenson, Robert Louis "The Lamplighter" 110–11
Tennyson, Lord Alfred "Ulysses" 113–14
"The Ladies on the Porch" 121–2
Wordsworth, William "I Wandered Lonely as a Cloud" 115–16
writing poems 120–6
Yeats, W.B. "The Song of Wandering Aengus" 124–6
positive language 36–7, 141–2
post-traumatic stress disorder (PTSD) 21–2
procedural memory system 28, 29–30
Psalms 150
putting something meaningful into someone's hands 143–4
connecting with the past 43, 49
recording stories 57
singing 98
video diaries 129, 136, 137
writing poems 120–1

Raichle, Marilyn 81–3
reading 55–7
    Esther's story 61
    games and exercises 62–8
    Georgia Dee's story 56
    Jenny's story 60
    Pat's story: Old Jewell 71–2
    Rebecca's story: the best gift
        69–70
    recording stories 56–61
    the pastor's story 58–9
    two reading circle stories 68–73
Renoir, Auguste *Dance at Bougival*
    80
Robinson, Sir Ken 76
Rose, Sitar 135–7
Round Table 86

semantic memory 29
singing 99–108
    choral singing 106–7
    Jackie's story 97–9
Sondheim, Stephen 108
Stevenson, Robert Louis 111
    "The Lamplighter" 110–11
stories, recording 57–61
    two reading circle stories 68–73
strength-based philosophies 18–19,
    33, 144

Tennyson, Lord Alfred "Ulysses"
    113–14
Thomas, Bill 47
Thomas, Dylan "A Child's
    Christmas in Wales" 78–9
Thoreau, Henry David 96
Tillich, Paul 45

veterans 46–7, 48–9
    Brenner, Tom 21–2
Vickhoff, Bjorn 107
video diaries 128–34
    Jo-Jo's story 127–8
    Marilyn's story 129
    Mary's story 132–3
    Paul's story 131
    using video diaries for training
        134–7

Wang, Laurie 134–5
Wordsworth, William 40, 115
    "I Wandered Lonely as a Cloud"
        115–16

Yeats, W.B. "The Song of
    Wandering Aengus" 124–6